On Our Terms

Empowering the New Health Consumer

GLEN TULLMAN

Todd Stansfield, Editor
Audra Gerber, Copy Editor

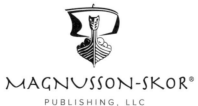

MAGNUSSON-SKOR®

PUBLISHING, LLC

Denver
www.mskor.com

Published by

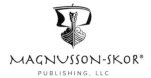

Magnusson-Skor Publishing
4600 S. Ulster Street Suite 1050
Denver, CO 80237
www.mskor.com

Library of Congress Control Number: 2018944195

Hardcover   ISBN 978-0-9998888-0-3
Paperback   ISBN 978-0-9998888-1-0

First Edition

*To a better health and health-care future . . .
one I know we can create and to the
leaders who will make it happen.*

" *Our greatest chance of solving the chronic-condition epidemic in
this country and across the world requires us to look to the last
place we might imagine: the person who is living with chronic
disease on a daily basis.*"

:: **Glen Tullman**, Author

CONTENTS

About the Author

Glen Tullman is the chairman and chief executive officer of Livongo Health. Livongo is empowering people with chronic conditions to live better and healthier lives. The company does this using a combination of innovative technology paired with personalized and context-sensitive information that is delivered when and where it is most impactful at improving health. While it all started with diabetes, today Livongo is the leading consumer digital-health company focusing on chronic conditions, including diabetes, hypertension, weight management, nutrition, and diabetes prevention. And by the time this goes to print, it may well include other chronic conditions because the company believes that to focus on health, you have to focus on the whole person, and that means addressing all of their health concerns.

A visionary leader and entrepreneur, Tullman previously led two public companies that changed the way health care is delivered. Most recently, he served as chief executive officer of Allscripts (NASDAQ: MDRX), a leading provider of electronic health records, practice management, and electronic prescribing systems, where during his tenure, he grew revenues from $30 million in 1997 to more than $1.4 billion in 2012 and led the company's initial public offering and secondary offerings. Prior to Allscripts, Tullman was chief executive officer of Enterprise Systems, which was at the time a leading health-care information services company that provided resource-management solutions to large, integrated health-care networks and hospital systems, which he also took public before it was sold to McKesson HBOC (NYSE: MCK).

Tullman is also cofounder and managing partner of 7wireVentures, a $100 million venture firm focused on early-stage health-care investing. Glen has founded or cofounded a number of ventures, including one of the country's leading commercial solar energy companies, SoCore Energy, sold to Edison Ventures, and a digital education company, now a part of Modern Teacher, and holds investments in several ventures focused on mobile and cloud-based health solutions. His broad interests range from ownership of Ignite Glass Studios in Chicago, one of the country's largest glass studios, to a major investment in Argo Tea, the largest independent tea company in the United States. Talk to him about his success and he'll immediately call out the people who surround him— longtime business partners Lee Shapiro and Joe Carey, who have been with him across many different businesses, and board members like Phil Green and Bob Compton, whom he names as mentors, investors, and most importantly, friends.

As a recognized leader in health care and entrepreneurship, Glen has been a contributor to *Forbes* and other leading publications, and is sought after as a speaker and industry expert on innovation and change. A strong proponent of philanthropy, he serves as a chancellor to the international board of the Juvenile Diabetes Research Foundation. Glen has three amazing children, all unique, and credits their mother, Trish, for giving them the grounding and balance to deal with his intensity.

Acknowledgments

This book would not have been possible without the encouragement of Charles Fred, the research and writing of Todd Stansfield, the editing of Lee Shapiro and Jennifer Schneider, and the constant support and ongoing education from my many partners, friends, and mentors, including Phil Green, Bob Compton, Hemant Taneja, Tom Main, Robert Garber, Joe Carey, and my executive leadership team at Livongo. And to Doug Candland, who taught me to write in the first place. The inspiration and good ideas are all theirs . . . the errors are all mine. And, of course, everything I do is driven by my desire to build a better world for Ben, Cayley, and Sam, who inspire me every day.

PREFACE

My real journey in truly understanding health care started in July 2003. My son Sam was diagnosed with Type 1 Diabetes. Sam was leading a pretty normal life with all the fun, challenges, and learning most eight-year-olds experience. He was visiting with his grandparents, and they noticed he was using the bathroom a lot—too much to be normal. So they took him to the pediatrician, and he was told he needed to be hospitalized immediately because he had Type 1 Diabetes.

Most people, especially today, have heard of diabetes but don't really understand it until they or someone they love is personally affected. There are two types of diabetes. Type 1, often called Juvenile Diabetes, is genetic. There is nothing you can do about it; you are born with it or it shows up, typically in the first 20 years of life, hence the name "juvenile." And historically, since kids didn't live all that long with it, it remained a juvenile disease. However, today there are more people alive with Type 1 Juvenile Diabetes over the age of 20 than under, due in large part to advances in how to treat and manage the disease. The second type of diabetes, called Type 2, has to do with lifestyle choices, including diet and exercise, and most commonly occurs over the age of 40, although because of the growing number of people who are overweight, especially in the United States, we're seeing that age drop and Type 2 appear in high school kids, particularly in under-resourced, inner-city settings.

Sam was labeled a "Type 1 Diabetic"—more on that later!

Both Sam's mother and I received the same call that neither of us will ever forget. Your son has diabetes. Nothing prepares you for that call . . . or any call about your child having a chronic disease. Then we were told that diabetes causes blindness and amputations, and typically kids with diabetes don't live as long as other "normal" kids—more on that later as well. Even today, as I type these words, my eyes still well up with tears. I was angry and sad, and honestly didn't know what to do other than to rush to his side. I jumped on a plane and was with him within hours. When I arrived at the hospital, I knew I needed to be strong for him so he wouldn't be scared. When you're the parent, your kids, while they don't always act like it, expect you to be the safety net. They want to be independent but want to know you are there to catch them when they fall, to clean up the scrapes and cuts, and to support them when life's challenges get in the way. So I shouldn't have been surprised when, after I walked into the room, Sam looked at me with his big blue eyes and said, "Dad, can you fix this?" I took the deepest breath I had ever taken and said confidently, "Yes." From that moment forward, my passion for finding a cure for diabetes, and helping people with diabetes stay healthy until we do, was ignited.

That scenario is played out every day in the United States

and around the world as parents are told their children have Type 1 Diabetes and, perhaps with just as much concern but less drama, as adults are told they have Type 2 Diabetes. We were fortunate for a sad reason. My brother Warren's daughter Ashley was diagnosed with Type 1 Diabetes just three years before, and we had become active in the Juvenile Diabetes Research Foundation (JDRF), the world's preeminent research organization focused on finding a cure. And we were already doing what good people do to support others facing any difficulty: we walked for a cure and attended fundraising galas, and I joined the local Chicago board of JDRF. And along the way, we learned about the disease. But nothing prepares you for the call, so when we received it, we at least knew that with proper support and care, people with Type 1 Diabetes could live normal and healthy lives.

And once you get over the emotional aspects of diabetes, you then realize the impact that diabetes has on the life of your son or daughter and the entire family. When Sam was diagnosed, there were no insulin pens, no connected technology, and very little to make living with diabetes manageable. So for many years, every night, either his mom or I had to wake up, wake him up, check his blood sugar, and get him to fall back asleep. For the first few years, there was never a night we slept through. And everyone needed to be educated on how to help Sam—school, camps (if they would take him, because some wouldn't), and coaches. Even a sleepover at a friend's house was an ordeal for Sam. And as we learned, some parents were too uncomfortable with the responsibility to invite him back. So we understood that this is life with diabetes—and how it would be from the day he was diagnosed until we find the elusive cure. This was our life.

Sam's life was one of pricking his finger about 10 times a day, every day. So many pricks that his fingers became callused. And writing down his blood sugar testing results. Remembering insulin. On hot days, having to keep the insulin cool. Visits to the endocrinologist and the school nurse. And all of that assuming the insurance company approved his strips, needles, and insulins, and didn't change them (which they did regularly if they could save a few dollars or get a larger rebate, having no sense of the impact on the people who use them). Imagine, as Sam has, pricking your finger more than 58,000 times. Imagine dealing with highs and lows (of blood sugar) that you can't control in the moment . . . at your most important moments . . . before the big exam, the SAT, the big game, the prom. Words can't capture the challenge and the bravery of these young kids and adults who manage this every day.

And all along, I was running software companies making every other aspect of life easier, more productive, safer. And I knew that we could do better. I knew we could make it easier to stay healthy; use software, technology, data science, and simple consumer-friendly techniques to remove the hassles;

and put people back in charge of their health, taking back some of the control of their lives that diabetes had stolen from them.

The good news is that Sam is doing well, and as every father or mother can understand, I'm very proud of him, especially given the extra challenges he's faced. But not every person with diabetes is so lucky.

Fast forward 10 years, my longtime business partner, Lee Shapiro, and I created an early-stage investment fund, pooling our funds and asking others to join, to look for opportunities that could make a meaningful difference in health and health care. The fund, named 7wireVentures (for the first transatlantic cable, which was seven copper wires, an innovation that transformed communications and commerce), took a unique and different view toward what we would invest in. We would invest in businesses that would help to create an "informed, connected health consumer." The idea was about any business that could

- make people better informed about their health and health-care decisions;
- not only get them connected to the cloud but get the cloud connected to them (like remote monitoring);
- focus on health—keeping people out of the hospital (preventive care); and
- treat people not as patients but as people or, more commercially, health consumers.

As a part of our search, we consulted Hemant Taneja, perhaps the brightest young tech investor in Silicon Valley, who was sent there by General Catalyst (the renowned Boston-based investment firm founded by David Fialkow and Joel Cutler) to establish a foothold and who has built an extraordinary investment portfolio. Hemant invited me out to meet with a few early-stage companies with a simple proposition: the weather is better in Silicon Valley than in Chicago, and we'll feed you. After looking at dozens of companies, we were introduced to a visionary mad scientist, inventor, and entrepreneur by some people who knew of my interest in diabetes. This entrepreneur had a working prototype of a cellular glucometer (the device used to check blood sugar by people with diabetes). While he knew and we knew he wasn't the right person to scale the company, we had a broader vision for a connected network that would begin with diabetes and would extend much further, eventually managing both health and health care.

As we looked at the company, and after many years of watching Sam deal with all the challenges, my sense was that the opportunity had arrived to change the care paradigm for people with diabetes, and my business partners said, "You have to do this!"

And I agreed. But I knew it couldn't be just about Sam. While Sam's personal experience allowed me to see, better understand, and experience the problem up close and personally, the big idea was about more than my son. It was the prospect of transforming and improving the experience and the lives of millions of people who struggle with diabetes, high blood pressure, weight, depression, behavioral health, and other chronic conditions every day. I understood in a very personal way how hard we make it for people to stay healthy. I just knew we could make it better—for everyone. And it all came together . . . *beshert*—a Yiddish word that means "it was meant to be."

I've been fortunate to have had a broad range of experiences that all served to prepare me to better understand both the challenges we face in health care today and the range of solutions available to us to truly empower people to live better and healthier lives. Let me mention a few. First, after more than 20 years running technology companies, one thing that I have learned is that it's not about the technology but rather the experience and change it enables. Value gets created only when we create change in a way that leads to better outcomes, and when we solve problems that consumers face.

I initially discovered this lesson in my role as president and chief operating officer of CCC Information Services, a claims management and services company serving the auto insurance and auto-body collision repair industries. CCC, founded by my brother Howard as Certified Collateral Corporation, started with a simple but important idea: to replace the Red Book and Blue Book used to value cars with real market information, an idea well before its time and one of the first practical applications of what we call "big data" today. We did that by inventorying every car lot in the country and actually finding the exact car that was a total loss due to an accident or a theft. After my brother left the business and went on to successfully start many others, we moved from locating and replacing cars to valuing cars, to providing collision estimates on cars and trucks, to managing the entire claims process, all by applying technology and information in innovative ways. Along the way, we ran into a few billion-dollar companies, like ADP, a legendary company and competitor at the time, and in every encounter, we beat them, with a lot of hustle, driven by the fear of not surviving, and a healthy dose of new technology and innovation. CCC Information Services went on to help Allstate, State Farm, Progressive, Geico, and many other customers reengineer their entire automobile claims processes, enabling "direct repair," which made the process of filing a claim and getting your damaged car or truck repaired much easier and more satisfying for consumers, with higher-quality repairs completed more quickly and at lower costs. In the beginning, both insurance-company and body-shop adjusters saw our computerized system as competition to their handwritten estimates. While they resisted our system initially, they soon embraced it after discovering that the technology made the entire process—writing the estimate, getting a rental car, ordering parts, and delivering a quality repair in a reasonable time—better for everyone.

Early on, we realized that we should only use technology if it can solve problems and improve our lives, and not because it simply represents something neat or something new. Technology didn't convince me to start a business improving how we manage chronic conditions. Understanding how hard we have made it for people, like my own son, to stay healthy was the impetus.

At Enterprise Systems, I was introduced to health care. ESI was in the business of resource management—that is, helping hospitals be more efficient and deliver better care. We pioneered checklists in the operating room to ensure that when someone was being operated upon, the entire medical team and all the necessary medical and surgical supplies were ready and in place. It all had to come together. What had previously operated in silos became one integrated team, and that led to better outcomes. This same challenge exists in health care today, especially with chronic conditions. Seventy percent of the people with diabetes also have other co-morbidities, like hypertension. In most cases, treating only one condition simply doesn't work, which is what led to our realization that only treating someone's diabetes wouldn't necessarily lead to a healthy person; we needed to be ready to treat the "whole person," which would include all their other conditions.

At Allscripts, where we pioneered electronic prescribing

at scale and then moved into practice management and, ultimately, into electronic medical records (alternatively known as EMRs and EHRs), we laid the foundation for better health care by making a patient's medical information available in digital form. EHRs were necessary but not a sufficient condition for improving health care. It has become increasingly clear today that EHRs are data repositories, and the new challenge is to use that electronic data and turn it into actionable information, provided at just the right time, to physicians and their patients, to truly improve health care.

So my journey—learning to use technology but not worship it as more than a means to an end, to understand process redesign and how silos inhibit successful outcomes, and finally, to recognize that having all the data in the world doesn't matter if you can't turn it into actionable information for the people who need it—has informed much of what you will read about in this book. My objective is to make the case for empowering people to live better and healthier lives by focusing on the whole person, not one part of them, and by leveraging technology-fueled solutions with a human touch.

Diabetes is the largest and fastest-growing chronic condition in the world, yet it is also the most manageable, but only if we give people information and the technology they need to manage it well. Most people with chronic conditions have more than one. So we understood early on that if we wanted to help people get healthy and stay healthy, we had to focus on the whole person and not look at chronic conditions in silos. And we decided to begin with diabetes.

Our work at Livongo is all about empowering people to live better and healthier lives—to live beyond their chronic condition. We have developed a proven methodology that achieves this aim—one validated by years of research, experience, and empirical evidence—and leads to effective and sustainable behavior change that results in people actually living better and healthier lives. We believe this is the ultimate solution to chronic conditions, and we use three metrics to prove it: user satisfaction, measurable clinical outcomes, and cost reduction. This book presents our methodology and research to help others discover a better pathway forward.

In the introduction of this book, we've presented the unique case studies of PepsiCo, Iron Mountain Incorporated, and WEA Trust, three organizations with separate stories of how they interact with the traditional health-care system. PepsiCo and Iron Mountain illustrate the challenge facing all businesses, but especially large and mid-sized self-insured employers. While they have a vested interest in the health of their employees and their families, and while they are, in large part, financially responsible for the costs of care, self-insured employers have to date been powerless to control health-care expenses beyond providing largely ineffective programs and tools their employees don't use.

Increasingly, the leading and most progressive of these

companies are taking matters into their own hands, going directly to new innovative companies outside the traditional health system to manage care and costs. PepsiCo and Iron Mountain are perfect examples, showing how self-insured employers are now offering more personalized solutions and actively engaging in open dialogue that encourages members to live better and healthier lives, all while maintaining the balance of the employer-employee relationship.

While this trend could easily leave payers behind, WEA Trust, a mid-sized payer headquartered in Wisconsin, is a great example of how the leading payers will also embrace innovation as a competitive strategy to improve quality, lower cost, and increase access to care.

All three organizations illustrate how innovation can drive better measurable outcomes, including user satisfaction, clinical outcomes, and financial measures, and should provide ample evidence that we can fix health care's challenges and do so today—reminding us of the quote that "the future is here; it's just not evenly distributed." These companies serve as examples that we can, with the right kind of leadership, make productive and important changes now.

Part one of this book explores the tyranny of the status quo—mainly, the rising cost and declining value of the health-care system as it grows more overwhelmed by a problem it fundamentally cannot solve. Today's health-care system remains designed to treat acute problems. In America, we're the best in the world at complex surgeries. For example, in heart surgery, we have come so far that people can be out of the hospital days after the most complex coronary bypass. Current medical advancements across a range of diseases are nothing short of amazing.

However, for chronic conditions—the kind that never go away—we're using the wrong tools in a system not designed to solve the problem. Rather than empower people with chronic conditions to live beyond the constraints of physicians and hospitals, the current solution attempts to "engage" people in an expensive, physician-driven model of care designed for acute conditions.

Once you understand what doesn't work and why, you can begin to appreciate new models enabling significant innovation and see the impact of an emerging and soon-to-be-dominant player in the mix: the "informed, connected health consumer." This emerging actor will no longer tolerate traditional health care's answer and is working to change the existing system through the power of the purse.

Part two of this book presents the solution to better address chronic conditions based on a model of empowerment. Unlike engagement, empowerment puts "informed, connected health consumers" in charge with everything they need to manage their condition. Empowerment recognizes that when people have access to quality information and tools, they are far more likely and capable of achieving and sustaining better health, all at lower costs, and that makes them happy campers.

Part three explores the empowerment model in depth, including the three essential components that make it possible. First, the model calls for empowering consumers with real-time information that is personalized, context aware, simple, and actionable. Second, it calls for enabling consumers to build their own caring community that understands their needs and can provide psychological and social support. Third, the model requires access to real-time care—typically provided by people, including some of the existing caregivers in the system today—delivered when and how people want it to stay healthy in the moment. We also explore the need for traditional players in the health-care system to adopt innovation as an imperative, and that includes everyone: health-care providers (both physicians and other caregivers on an individual level and hospitals on a system level), pharmacy benefit managers (PBMs), and pharmaceutical companies.

This book presents an effective and sustainable solution to dealing with chronic conditions. Why not empower the people with the greatest influence to drive better outcomes? Why not invest in treating the source of the problem—behavior— rather than treating its symptoms: complications, expensive hospital visits, and other collateral effects? To truly address the chronic-care epidemic calls for shifting responsibility to a participant who, up until now, has taken a passive role in the health-care system. But today, that is changing. The "informed, connected health consumer" will replace the "passive patient" in our traditional health-care system. And rather than fight this change, we must embrace it, support it, and fuel it.

ON
OUR
TERMS

Empowering the
New Health Consumer

INTRODUCTION

"The best way out is always through."

—Robert Frost

In 1997, the World Health Organization released its world health report titled "Conquering Suffering, Enriching Humanity."[1] The report focused on chronic conditions and predicted they would become a global epidemic in the next two decades. Today, that prediction holds true. Chronic conditions are the leading cause of death worldwide. In the United States alone, chronic conditions account for 70 percent of deaths and consume the majority of health-care spending.[2] This trend will only accelerate—not because our health-care system is failing but rather because it is designed to solve a different problem: it provides treatment of acute problems, not prevention. The health-care system of the future will need to focus on <u>predicting</u> health-care issues before they happen, <u>prescribing</u> the right solutions—which may have little to do with traditional health care—and <u>preventing</u> bad outcomes and the costs associated with them. While we won't eliminate all chronic conditions, we will delay onset and better manage them when they do occur. The "we" turns out to be each of us, with a system that makes it easier to stay healthy in the first place and then treat conditions in the best way possible.

Precisely for that reason, we can see a movement that is not being driven by those operating the health-care system but by those dependent upon it. For the first time, these stakeholders are now driving change outside the status quo, recognizing

[1] *The world health report 1997 - conquering suffering, enriching humanity*, (Geneva: The World Health Organization, 1997), http://www.who.int/whr/1997/en/.
[2] "Chronic Disease Prevention and Health Promotion," Centers for Disease Control and Prevention, last modified December 18, 2017, https://www.cdc.gov/chronicdisease/index.htm.

that the real risk is not taking a chance on change but doing nothing, which maintains the status quo. Fortunately, several pioneering organizations are forging a new pathway forward, signaling the beginning of a broader shift to address chronic conditions more cost effectively and sustainably in the future.

Traditional players in the health-care space are not moving quickly enough, so self-insured employers—who are paying the bills—are stepping in to introduce all kinds of new innovation. PepsiCo, one of the leading food and beverage companies in the world, serves as a good example. With medical costs rising at an unacceptable rate, PepsiCo sought a new path for the approximately 190,000 participants in its health plan.[3] Seeing that employees with chronic conditions (who account for the majority of health-care spending) lacked access to programs that provided the information and tools to better manage their own health, PepsiCo chose to face a challenge universally shared by all large self-insured employers head-on. It owned the responsibility for managing the health-care costs of its members, yet it lacked direct control to reduce spending by offering programs that members would value and would feel motivated to participate in. PepsiCo's largest health-care expenditures came from participants with multiple chronic conditions, which are largely manageable through healthier lifestyle behaviors. Improving health and thus lowering costs would mean convincing these participants

---

[3]"6 Lessons from Pepsi on Engaging Employees beyond Workplace Wellness." *Engaging Leader*. April 28, 2016. Accessed September 13, 2017. http://www.engagingleader.com/6-lessons-from-pepsi/.

to adopt new behaviors, yet this remained a delicate matter, as employees typically see their health as outside the purview of their employer. As a public company with a responsibility to shareholders and stakeholders as well as its employees, PepsiCo sought an innovative solution that would encourage members to adopt healthier habits, alleviating the cost burden while improving clinical results and satisfaction. Ultimately, the corporation sought to foster a new relationship with employees, where they viewed PepsiCo as a partner in their path to living better and healthier lives.

Iron Mountain, the global leader in storage and information management services, faced similar challenges. Its health-care costs were rising at an average annual rate of 11 percent, above national averages. Entering 2013, the Boston, Massachusetts-based enterprise faced a cost increase of over 12 percent. With an annual business growth rate in the United States of less than half that, Iron Mountain could not continue to support the increasing expense to cover more than 16,000 participants covered by its health plan. The cost increases were largely due to the poor clinical outcomes of participants with chronic conditions. For this group, Iron Mountain discovered that only 30 to 40 percent were consistently managing their conditions. The lack of engagement not only contributed significant increased costs to the health plan but also continued to drive related financial costs through presenteeism, absenteeism, and reduced productivity.

The story was similar at WEA Trust, a nonprofit insurance company that serves public employers, which means their health care is paid for directly by taxpayers throughout Wisconsin. Not surprisingly, they also identified that the unsustainable growth in health-care costs they were experiencing were driven primarily by chronic illnesses. Their goal—to trim at least 16 percent in premium costs—would require helping members with chronic conditions significantly change their behaviors by better understanding their underlying illness, measuring it, and sharing this information with their care community. For the communities WEA served living below the poverty level, the payer focused on making health insurance affordable to populations by encouraging less unplanned, uncoordinated care and assuring that members were directly participating in their own health decisions.

Fortunately, changes from Washington helped create an environment more conducive for new approaches. The Patient Protection and Affordable Care Act (ACA) of 2009 initiated a fundamental movement that among other things, made people more financially responsible—by significantly increasing deductibles—for a meaningful portion of their annual health-care premiums. The growth of high-deductible health plans (HDHPs) and health savings accounts (HSAs) led to behaviors and expectations previously unseen in the traditional health-care system. While many people viewed these changes as government intervention, or on a more extreme level, a government takeover of health care, the reality is that the ACA drove millions of patients to become health consumers. For the first time in health care, people began to act like consumers, demanding value for what they now needed to pay for. They expected more positive experiences and responsive, personalized service found in other aspects of their lives, and they wanted tools and information that provided them with autonomy, transparency, convenience, and control in the management of their health.

PepsiCo seized this moment to foster a new dialogue with employees. While employees traditionally view health as beyond the interest of their employers, their new financial responsibility made them more receptive to PepsiCo's involvement. Frankly, just as their employers had done, they realized that the increasing costs of health care were unsustainable, and they were ready and willing to take help from anyone—including their employers. As members sought to understand how to better control their costs, PepsiCo communicated the need for members to see the value—both physical and financial—of managing their health. The company also defined its role and interest in helping members achieve better outcomes, and with that came PepsiCo's commitment to giving members the best tools in the marketplace. In doing so, PepsiCo positioned itself as a partner in the journey toward better health, a sustainable position where the company could actively encourage and support members, while nurturing a culture that emphasized healthy behaviors.

With employees now on board, PepsiCo sought to find new innovative programs. It approached the marketplace with a guiding thesis: all programs should treat employees as health consumers and offer them personalized, real-time solutions. A consumer approach would mean enabling members to drive the experience and gain access to all the needed tools and information to manage their health independently. Personalized health care would call for treating members as unique individuals rather than as one similar group—the latter being a consistent approach for traditional programs. Requiring real time would necessitate 24/7 access and availability wherever needed. This approach would ease the burden of managing a chronic condition significantly. By making it easier to access programs uniquely tailored to their needs, members would be more satisfied and drive better health, at lower costs.

At about the same time, in 2013, Iron Mountain began aggressively investing in new and emerging solutions. Most of these programs shared the fundamental characteristics of increasing the personalization, accessibility, and availability of health care. For participants with metabolic syndrome— generally defined as a cluster of conditions including high blood pressure, high blood sugar, unhealthy cholesterol levels, and high levels of abdominal fat—Iron Mountain began offering a variety of programs: a platform through Omada Health, based on prior studies on diabetes prevention, that provided participants with programs to delay or prevent the onset of Type 2 Diabetes. For those people with diabetes, Iron Mountain also began providing Livongo, my own company's program, to better understand, manage, connect with a personal community, and gain access to real-time, context-sensitive care. Additionally, the company provided employees resilience training through meQuilibrium for mental health and stress management. For participants with chronic obstructive pulmonary disease (COPD) and congestive heart failure, Iron Mountain also introduced a program that leveraged self-diagnostic technology, cloud-based technology, and remote support.

While PepsiCo and Iron Mountain were offering a slew of new programs, WEA Trust committed to the member being in control of sharing his or her information and seeking additional trusted guidance outside of traditional health care. The sharing of clinical data and cost information to members revealed itself as the only viable solution to improve health while, at the same time, managing costs in a meaningful way. This strategy would focus on accelerating new member-focused information-sharing programs while, at the same time, redesigning how WEA could leverage its large number of lives to move care toward providers who shared this vision.

For these organizations, taking action and showing early leadership in redefining how they approached health and health care not only paid dividends for their employees' health and their bottom line but also served to support the new innovative companies providing the necessary services. This new direction required a new approach with employees, members, and insured stakeholders, fundamentally redesigning mental models and systems, and securing new partners providing solutions that could address the broad and diverse needs of their respective populations. The fact that three distinct organizations all realized the need to change signaled a turning point for the status quo and is a trend that is accelerating.

Consider where PepsiCo stands today. Long recognized for being a health-minded and employee-oriented organization, PepsiCo has developed a comprehensive suite of programs aimed to identify, prevent, and treat chronic conditions for its members—sounding similar to Livongo's predict, prescribe, and prevent methodology. Central to these programs is first understanding members' needs (and the requisite data and information required) and the commitment to personalized attention and support. With members now more aware of the financial impact of their health, these programs take a consumer-oriented approach, not only focusing on providing better information and tools to promote health but also creating an experience members value. There is an implicit

9

assumption, also common to Livongo's way of thinking, that if you make it easy to stay healthy, people will take advantage of anything you offer.

PepsiCo has worked to make it easy to learn about and access these programs. For example, its Health ACE Program connects members to appropriate health programs for their health issues and answers any of their questions—from administration to benefits to managing a certain condition. Members can call a dedicated team member to gain access to a live professional trained in all the programs PepsiCo offers. These professionals, often referred to as navigators, connect members to the right programs that reflect their actual needs.

Another example is PepsiCo's use of Livongo, which employs remote patient monitoring to empower members with personalized insights and suggestions, the ability to create and access their own caring community, and real-time 24/7 care for their chronic conditions. PepsiCo also offers an employee assistance program, which provides 24/7 support from trained behavioral-science professionals. All of PepsiCo's programs share a focus on providing members with the tools and information they need to manage their health, when they need it, and puts them in charge, allowing them to choose the program that is most relevant to them.

Additionally, the company takes a personalized approach to how it communicates programs. Rather than announce all programs to all members, the company leverages internal and external data insights to send targeted communications to the right members at the right time after they opt in. For example, PepsiCo sends a message about proper management of asthma when pollen counts reach a high level, given the increased risk for the condition to flare up during those times. The message isn't sent to all 190,000 participants (which includes employees and their covered family members)—only to people who have the condition, live in the affected area, and are at risk at the time. This approach ensures members gain value from the communication, increasing the likelihood of using it while, at the same time, not tuning out messages.

Due to these efforts, PepsiCo continues to see impressive results in the health and engagement of its members. It now sees strong and steady improvement in measures that indicate people are better managing their conditions. PepsiCo also sees an improvement in the satisfaction of members, particularly those with chronic conditions. And PepsiCo continues to maintain a lower cost of health insurance than its peers through active management and support of its members beyond traditional doctors' visits.

Iron Mountain has achieved similar results. After going live with its new programs in 2014, the annual trend of rising health-care costs fell to 2.4 percent. This marked a significant achievement, especially since the organization did not make significant changes to the design of its health plan. Today, Iron Mountain's health-plan costs consistently fall below the national benchmarks associated with health-care expenses. Iron Mountain also continues to see improvements in the clinical results and satisfaction of its participants. Iron Mountain conducted a two-year study focused on two populations with diabetes—one with access to the Livongo diabetes solution and a control group without access—and measured the impact of personalized, real-time insights and access that empowered people to live healthier on their terms. The conclusion was that the population using Livongo cut health-care expenses by 3 percent, while the latter saw a 14 percent annual increase in costs. The population using Livongo also saw inpatient and emergency room (ER) admissions decrease by 54 and 40 percent, respectively. Most important, however, was an increase in both compliance and satisfaction from employees and dependents.

Iron Mountain continues to strengthen its commitment around innovation, understanding the value of providing employees and dependents with better, more timely information and access to care, and doing so in a personalized way. Currently, Iron Mountain is going live with a digital navigation platform offered by Evive. The platform builds unique profiles for each of its members and provides information and notifications tailored to their specific needs. For example, the platform sends personalized communications through text and email, so participants understand how to better manage their health and gain access to programs they need and want. In another preemptive move, Iron Mountain plans to provide free genetic testing to participants to identify people with higher genetic risk factors for chronic conditions, such as cancer, that are impacted by lifestyle behaviors. The program addresses lifestyle behaviors that ultimately lead to preventable chronic conditions and give people options to begin to modify behaviors. To remain on the cutting edge, Iron Mountain participates in Mercer's Annual Healthcare Innovation Symposium, which showcases the innovations of early-stage companies in health care. This is another example of Iron Mountain's commitment to scaling new innovations for people covered by its health plan, ensuring they gain access to more personalized, available, and accessible health care. Iron Mountain is a true innovator and doesn't wait until the market has worked through every aspect of the program. Their view, simply stated, is that health care is too big an issue to wait for and that it's important to lead the way.

13

WEA Trust also found dramatic improvements in clinical and financial results from actively and aggressively innovating in the health space. The Wisconsin payer offers a variety of programs designed to personalize care to members. Like PepsiCo and Iron Mountain, WEA Trust offers programs that provide expert navigation to members when and where they need help. Patients who receive a cancer diagnosis are immediately assigned a navigation specialist who can guide them through their entire experience, focusing on getting the diagnosis right, matching the treatment, and reducing predictable unplanned care, like treatment for nausea and vomiting. The WEA Trust member service call line guarantees members can access a member specialist within 30 seconds of calling, underscoring its commitment to taking a consumer-oriented approach. Recognizing the lack of behavioral-health services in the state, it also offers members a convenient and affordable behavioral-telehealth platform, which provides support for participants taking antidepressants or suffering with mental-health issues. This program not only provides access whenever and wherever it's needed, solving the problem of access and availability, but also eliminates the stigma and patient disclosure that happen when visiting a physical location. The program ensures people feel encouraged to receive the care they need.

WEA Trust has also taken their commitment to innovation a step further than all but the largest payers with their recent investment in a Wisconsin-based health-care technology company providing, among other things, a platform that helps people with back pain gain access to real-time, personalized care and avoid opiates. The idea of a payer getting into the venture business can be scary but also speaks to the urgent need for solutions. The consistent message from the best companies is, they are no longer waiting for the market for solutions; they will actually help invent solutions, or partner and fund innovations if they can unlock better experiences and outcomes for their members. Currently, WEA Trust, like other larger payers, also serves as an advisor to and limited partner of Venture Investors, a Madison-based venture-capital group that funds early-stage enterprises creating innovations in health care. Essentially, WEA Trust has created a model to drive continual innovation, one that is market—not government—driven. This unique approach ensures WEA Trust can continue innovating to stay on the leading but not bleeding edge.

The results speak for themselves. WEA Trust continues to see improvement in clinical results, member satisfaction, and financial results. The company has cut costs by 16 percent while maintaining one of the lowest complaint rates in Wisconsin for any state or national health insurer.

So what can we learn from PepsiCo, Iron Mountain, and WEA Trust? All three have taken unique approaches to address the same fundamental problem. In fact, this challenge is universally shared by every entity involved in our health-care system, including large self-insured employers, payers, health-care providers, and pharmacy benefit managers (PBMs). It stems from a growing epidemic that promises to worsen in the future: chronic conditions. Their rapid proliferation continues to expose the flaws of our current health-care system, which is designed to address a far different kind of problem than the type that never goes away.

Pioneers like PepsiCo, Iron Mountain, and WEA Trust are uncovering a new way forward based on innovation and action—putting new solutions into practice. This is a model others can follow. And all three companies have learned that to demonstrate better outcomes requires a systematic approach toward innovation that puts health consumers at the center. It begins with providing them everything they need to manage their health on their terms and not on ours, and it is the best answer we have to solving the chronic-condition epidemic.

Part I:

The Tyranny of the
Status Quo

CHAPTER 1:
MAKING THE CASE FOR A NEW APPROACH

" If you want something new, you have to stop doing something old. "

The health-care system is designed to treat problems that have a transactional cure. And the system—a vast and interconnected network of patients, providers, payers, medical schools, hospitals, and other entities—operates according to a model crafted around places rather than the digital ecosystem we live in today. This model encompasses the entire process, from providing and receiving treatment to getting paid for its delivery. Despite challenges from a cost and quality perspective—which are considerable—the health-care system works when fixing a broken arm, treating a sinus infection or performing complex heart surgery.

Unfortunately, the health-care needs of the world population have shifted at an accelerated rate over the past few decades. Conditions such as diabetes, heart disease, and depression have become pervasive, requiring fundamentally different solutions than those applied in the world of acute care. Two shifts are occurring: the first is a change in the problem we need to solve, and the second is a change in the people we are treating—they have become digital consumers. The traditional health-care system is designed to treat transactional problems, where a patient enters the health-care system, receives treatment, and leaves. That's a fundamentally different problem to solve than someone who must manage a chronic condition for the rest of his or her life. The move toward a digital consumer means we need a new set of tools to treat them and have a new set of expectations to meet. The past successes of the health-care system—extending life and treating acute conditions—now obstruct its own ability to evolve and address chronic conditions effectively. Inertia, resulting from a status quo of the previous design, serves as a perpetual constricting force. For example, medical schools are designed to train clinicians to perform surgical procedures, not to enable people with heart disease to live healthier, more productive lives and prevent the need for the surgery in the first place. That has not changed. It turns out that this is mostly about system design (often called population health) versus individual cures. Acute-care facilities, while equipped to handle the most challenging cases from a medical care standpoint, lack the resources and capacity to adequately supply the services and

"Inertia, resulting from a status quo of the previous design, serves as a perpetual constricting force."

around-the-clock care that a population with diabetes or hypertension needs.

The more important question, though, is this: should hospitals even try? Even the most universal clinical innovations remain designed for acute practice. A stethoscope provides basic measurement of whether patients are alive at that moment. More sophisticated technology, such as MRI, captures a picture of health at a current point in time. Neither provides the continuous measurement of health that people with chronic conditions need—including how they live and experience life—and that all of us will soon want. Today, more than 60 percent of Americans suffer from a chronic condition.[4] More than 30 million Americans suffer from Type 1 or Type 2 Diabetes alone, and it wins the title as the fastest-growing chronic condition in the world. In the next 10 years, more people in China and India will have diabetes than the entire US population. The rise of chronic disease is precipitous, and our focus on acute care and everything that surrounds it remains far too ingrained and systemic to respond appropriately to the rapid increase in chronic disease. People, infrastructure, payment models, and

> "People, infrastructure, payment models, and incentives are neither aligned nor ready for the change."

---

[4] Christine Buttorff, Teague Ruder, and Melissa Bauman, *Multiple Chronic Conditions in the United States*, (Santa Monica: RAND Corporation, 2017), 6.

incentives are neither aligned nor ready for the change. Even if people were ready to adopt them, there are very few tools to comprehensively manage a population—predicting who will need care and prescribing the appropriate care in order to prevent complications in the first place. For people with ongoing health conditions, the system continues to

> **"We are seeing the beginning of this implosion today."**

accept them, provide episodic treatment, and bill them as if they are cured of their conditions.

So what happens when the system, upon which so many depend, must evolve? When the acute-care facility must treat conditions that never go away? When those entering the system need more time and attention than health-care professionals can devote? When the system's episodic design—processes, structures, mental models, relationships—no longer remains tenable? It implodes. We are seeing the beginning of this implosion today. Health-care costs continue to skyrocket at an unsustainable rate, with chronic conditions accounting for nearly nine out of every ten dollars spent.[5] Even as expenditures rise, quality of care and patient outcomes continue to decline, underscoring the systemic nature and extent of the problem. Meanwhile, health-care providers continue to grapple with a

21

---

[5] "At a Glance 2015," *National Center for Chronic Disease Prevention and Health Promotion,* accessed September 13, 2017, https://www.cdc.gov/chronicdisease/resources/publications/aag/pdf/2015/nccdphp-aag.pdf

shortage of resources in the wake of rising demand, and self-insured employers and patients continue to assume more cost and risk from an overpriced, overburdened system of care.

Simply put, the health-care system as it is currently designed cannot supply the time and attention needed to address chronic conditions. Currently, people with chronic conditions are responsible for managing 99.9 percent of their health issues without access to good information or the support they need when they need it. If even a fraction of people living with a chronic condition simultaneously tried to access the system, it would be overwhelmed—there simply aren't enough physicians to meet the demand as defined today. The key is "as defined today." Even if we wanted to address diabetes, we would have a shortage of clinical knowledge and capacity. The average physician only receives a few days of clinical practice in nutrition,[6] which is essential to managing diabetes and other chronic conditions. There are only 6,500 active endocrinologists currently practicing in the United States, or one for every 4,600 people fighting diabetes.[7] Given the current demand

> "Even if we wanted to address diabetes, we would have a shortage of clinical knowledge and capacity."

---

[6] Kelly Adams, W. Scott Butsch, and Martin Kohlmeier, "The State of Nutrition Education at US Medical Schools," *Journal of Biomedical Education* 2015 (August 2015), 3, http://dx.doi.org/10.1155/2015/357627 https357627, https://www.hindawi.com/journals/jbe/2015/357627/

[7] *2014 Physician Specialty Physician Data Book.* (Washington, DC: Association of Medical Colleges, June 3, 2015), 15.

for physicians, we simply can't solve the problem with more physicians (it would take too long to produce them and cost too much). What we need is a different approach. So what happens when the system must evolve? If it doesn't, it implodes.

The health-care system, including physicians, hospitals, and payers, universally talk about the importance of engaging people in their health, yet the current approach toward truly engaging the patient in better health outcomes and lifestyle changes remains essentially inadequate. Patient engagement strategies—a collection of initiatives, programs, and innovations designed to increase compliance with treatment decisions—tend to focus on ways of force-fitting people into solutions that simply don't work well or provide value. For

instance, traditional disease management programs try to increase participation in predesigned care plans by calling at home or at work, reminding patients they have a

"In most cases, the disease management program is designed for the care provider, not for the nuance of daily life with a chronic illness."

condition, and asking if they need help, a practice patients universally despise. Patient portals—providing access to electronic health records to improve efficiency, while not addressing cost—aim to inform and educate by giving patients electronic access to test results and the ability to message their provider, but few patients access them. In most cases, the disease management program is designed for the care provider, not for the nuance of daily life with a chronic illness. For example, contact is made when most convenient for the provider, not for the patient. The patient portal, though delivering the electronic message, still cannot convey a response until the provider sends one. The approach forces people to become more reliant on a provider-centric system that cannot supply the time, provide the resources, or engender the behaviors to appropriately manage chronic conditions.

How does the health-care system need to change to accommodate those living with chronic conditions? The present health-care system cannot evolve fast enough to address the chronic-condition crisis. The country now stands at a critical inflection point where individuals fighting chronic conditions must take charge of their health and stop relying on a system that invariably limits their knowledge and control. The kind of change the nation needs—sustainable and scalable across populations—starts with serving health-care consumers on *their* terms and utilizing technology that is capable of empowering them. We

"We have to realize that like every other industry, health care is an information business."

have to realize that like every other industry, health care is an information business. Truly better outcomes depend on what these consumers can learn and understand about their health patterns, and the lifestyle behaviors and conditions that influence them. The more information they gain, the more knowledge they acquire, the more confidence they attain, and the more likely they develop and reinforce habits that lead to better health outcomes. No solution is more scalable than one that empowers the resource capable of making a difference and guaranteed to be in adequate supply. No solution is more sustainable than one that truly addresses the core problem—lifestyle behaviors—that causes most chronic conditions. The answer to addressing chronic conditions is one that also empowers individuals' support network of family and friends—the most influential resource available to offer assistance and encouragement—to understand how and when to offer the care that truly produces better outcomes. The solution also must connect those affected to the support they need from professionals specialized in their condition, but only when appropriate and in ways that make sense from a care and cost standpoint. This approach is far different from the current model but far more effective at giving people with chronic conditions the power and support they need to take charge and live beyond the shadow of their illness.

Technology can empower individuals affected by chronic conditions to treat their condition as a pattern of daily activities and behaviors rather than a random collection of episodes. Up until now, *the body's vital narrative*—the ongoing story of one's health—has remained a mystery. Sensors, smart-connected devices, and access to the power of the cloud to turn this data into information provide the only path to truly expand knowledge of chronic conditions and empower everyone in the health-care equation. People with chronic conditions can now learn how patterns of behavior affect their health and receive personalized, actionable, simple, and context-aware information to improve it. Delivered in real time and tailored uniquely to them, this real-time communication has the power to create the kind of new knowledge, confidence, and motivation absent today. Individuals can also gain access to support when they need it most. Professionals specialized in chronic conditions can provide around-the-clock support remotely, contacting people needing assistance only at the appropriate moment, a model that serves as the "OnStar"[8] for chronic-condition management. Additionally, family members and friends can overcome a sense of powerlessness by receiving alerts when, but only when, their support is needed and at the request and with the permission of the person with the chronic condition. Health-care providers can also optimize their resources to provide the right level of care at the right time, focusing on and getting paid for those patients who truly would benefit from professional care

[8] OnStar Corporation is a subsidiary of General Motors that provides in-vehicle technology to support drivers.

while rewarding individuals who are healthy with the extra time they get from not having to see a doctor for the routine checkup that can now be completed remotely. Self-insured employers, payers, health systems, and anyone else who owns the risk of paying for chronic conditions can better control health-care spending and reap the benefits of a healthier, more productive population.

These innovations exist not only to manage and improve chronic conditions but to prevent their most debilitating effects. It's not just a technology. It's rethinking the entire experience from a consumer-centric, digital-health perspective. Smart technology, coupled with data science, has unleashed the ability to enable entire populations to better manage their health, **predicting** who will need attention and care; **prescribing** what is the "right" care from a clinical, lifestyle, and cost standpoint for each individual; and most importantly, **preventing** or delaying chronic conditions in the first place.

"Nothing is more vital than people's health."

Health care is one of the last industries to leverage technology to become more efficient, effective, and productive, yet it remains the most important sector in our lives and for the economy. Nothing is more vital than people's health, because when they are sick, nothing else matters, and when loved ones are ill, it disrupts every aspect of our lives.

What can the health-care system do now to rewrite the *body's vital narrative* for the millions of people dealing with chronic conditions? How can it move from a model focused on "patient engagement" to one centered on "health-consumer empowerment"? These are critical questions in need of answers. This is one of the most important and immediate needs of our time. Success depends on whether all stakeholders of the health-care system can collectively unite—as leaders and participants—to embrace innovations capable of empowering people to take charge of their own health and make a sustainable impact in our collective fight against chronic conditions.

• • •

Chapter Summary

- "Conditions such as diabetes, heart disease, and depression have become pervasive, requiring fundamentally different solutions than those applied in the world of acute care. Two shifts are occurring: the first is a change in the problem we need to solve, and the second is a change in the people we are treating—they have become digital consumers."

- "The kind of change the nation needs—sustainable and scalable across populations—starts with serving healthcare consumers on *their* terms and utilizing technology that is capable of empowering them."

- "Smart technology, coupled with data science, has unleashed the ability to enable entire populations to better manage their health, **predicting** who will need attention and care; **prescribing** what is the 'right' care from a clinical, lifestyle, and cost standpoint for each individual; and most importantly, **preventing** or delaying chronic conditions in the first place."

29

CHAPTER 2:
INTRODUCING THE INFORMED CONNECTED
HEALTH CONSUMER

❝ *In a fight between you and the world, bet on the world."*

:: Franz Kafka

The passage of the Patient Protection and Affordable Care Act (ACA) initiated a monumental shift in the health-care system. Universal access to health care; a greater focus on improving the quality, accessibility, and affordability of care; and greater financial responsibility for employers and individuals all shifted the industry's center of gravity toward a model focused on value-based solutions and prevention for populations. While the future of the law remains unknown, many of its core elements will persist. It turns out that one of the key learnings was not that people don't want more health care but rather that they simply don't like paying for it. That said, all of the participants in the health-care equation— including political partisans—recognize the unsustainability of the current system. The transition from fee-for-service to pay-for-performance—tying reimbursement to improvements in clinical outcomes—represents a dramatic departure from the current system's design but is slow in coming. But the need for a new solution that drives consumer satisfaction and clinical quality, and slows the cost curve is as necessary as ever. This need is driving broad consolidations between and among diverse stakeholders, all to better coordinate care, leverage capabilities, achieve economies of scale, and manage the

"Simply providing a service no longer counts."

health of populations. Tomorrow will not depend on whether a pharmaceutical company can produce a profitable drug or sell it but whether it can ensure the proper use of the drug with the intended effect of both improving health and reducing overall system costs. In every way, the health-care system of tomorrow raises the bar on the requirements stakeholders take for granted today. Simply providing a service no longer counts. Performance—in the form of measurable outcomes and better care—matters, and everyone will share in the accountability for improving it. Silos will need to disappear. A surgeon who performs excellent surgery won't get his or her full reimbursement unless the rehab is successful in returning the patient to the original or better state of health.

31

The turbulence created by the ACA has led to the emergence of a new and increasingly powerful player in the health-care equation: the informed, connected health consumer. While many people argue that Obamacare was pushing government control of health care, the reality is that it created a new market with nearly 11.8 million consumers who were—for approximately the first $5,000 or more of health-care expenses—spending their own money.[9] Only now are we starting to see the kind of change this will drive. The informed, connected health consumer behaves much differently than the patient who once tolerated a lack of information and control, demanding transparency, affordability, and choice, and possessing the power of the purse—all borne out of new financial responsibility and access to better, more comprehensive information.

Let's define exactly what we mean by "informed, connected health consumers": **"Informed"** means having access to quality and timely information on cost, quality, availability, and options, which was previously unavailable to either patients or their physicians. **"Connected"** means not just connected to the internet, which drives this instant availability, but the internet connected to you, as a person and a patient, constantly monitoring your health state (also known as "remote patient monitoring"). This falls into the general trend of IOT or the Internet of Things, where everything is connected. So why not us? With remote patient monitoring, you're connected to the cloud, but the real value begins when the data analytics in the cloud give you the ability to monitor your own health. In fact, the terminology of "remote patient monitoring" is wrong. No one remotely monitors when you need to take an aspirin. A

---

[9] Alonso-Zaldivar, Ricardo, and Kevin S. Vineys. "AP Count: Nearly 11.8M Enroll for Obama Health Law in 2018." *AP News*. February 07, 2018. Accessed May 29, 2018. https://www.apnews.com/837a78792b9449 37b6e0fca69ee55e4e/AP-count:-Nearly-11.8M-enroll-for-Obama-health-law-in-2018.

better term is "self-monitoring and sharing," empowering you using devices and sensors to monitor your own health and informing you and others when you need assistance in some way. In the future, you won't schedule an appointment or visit a physician for a quarterly checkup. Rather, the system will evaluate your needs, your patterns, and compare your unique narrative to other people like you and recommend when you need to have lab tests or see a physician and then provide the most convenient, cost-effective options, which will drive much more efficient utilization of a precious and expensive resource: physicians.

"Health" refers to the fact that the goal is to keep people out of the health-care system and healthy. In quality parlance, when someone needs health care, that will be an error versus what we expect. And when people do need medical attention, the goal will be to triage them to the most effective, high-quality care that is also cost efficient (which generally will not be a physician) and treat them outside the four walls of the hospital. The goal will be

33

> **"In quality parlance, when someone needs health care, that will be an error versus what we expect."**

treatment at home, then at a convenient, local pharmacy ("take two of these and don't call me in the morning"), and then at a physician's office. Managing people outside the four walls of the hospital is important because the hospital and ER turn out to be the most expensive and resource-consuming part of our health-care system, and the most dangerous for secondary infections and other life-threatening challenges. Hospitals should be a last resort. Specialized, lower-cost, and more focused surgi-centers will perform most same-day surgeries with measurably better quality, fewer infections, and higher customer satisfaction. We will create models where we reward keeping people healthy in the first place and not fixing them. Health, not health care, is our goal.

"Consumers" refers to the fact that we are better off treating people like consumers rather than patients, whom we've trained to expect not to pay for services. Where we find that health services have been consumerized, quality tends to be higher, people are more satisfied, and the costs follow more of a traditional business curve—they fall with competition and over time. As a bonus, health consumers are willing to and expect to pay for these "consumerized" services.

"This necessary shift has produced behaviors well recognized in other industries."

So we now are developing a growing group of informed, connected health consumers. What will be their impact? While the ACA increased access to health insurance for consumers, it also increased their financial responsibility.

This necessary shift has produced behaviors well recognized in other industries. Forced to pay out of their own pockets, the new informed, connected health consumers will demonstrate greater scrutiny when it comes to their health care as they increasingly comparison shop among services and evaluate their experiences in relation to those of other sectors. The emergence of this new kind of health consumer has led to a watershed moment that will increasingly call into question why the system cannot provide the same information and service experience as today's most forward-thinking and innovative enterprises—such as Amazon, Uber, Apple, and less well-known companies like Zeel, which locates massage therapists and sends them to your home on demand, and TalkSpace, which provides mental health support—who combine digital smarts with services in ways that increase satisfaction, demand, and a willingness to pay!

35

The rise of the health consumer has also led to a greater push for innovation in a sector notoriously resistant to new technology. Only recently did health-care providers begin to universally adopt electronic health records (EHRs), and the process was slow, expensive, and painful for all involved. While EHRs have begun to lay the necessary foundations for an information-empowered industry, they are not sufficient. In fact, most of the EHRs today are simply data repositories that communicate the information entered into them, albeit in more legible and portable formats. However, the real value to be gained from EHRs will come from the analysis of their vast stores of data and the personalized recommendations they generate for physicians and the patients they are treating based on deep data science. The question remains whether the existing players—including Cerner, which is farthest along the path to next-generation information systems; Athena, which is one of the most innovative; and Allscripts, my former company—can or will make the leap. Epic, which enjoys significant share among large and well-known academic medical centers (which also tend to be the highest-cost delivery systems), is the farthest from the interoperable architecture and system design that will be required in the future. Today, EHR systems need a better front-end design of their user interface, which includes physician and patient input, as well as a back-end redesign, which will need to be more focused on information and insights than billing, which may, in the new world, disappear.

> "Today, EHR systems need a better front-end design of their user interface."

Today, the level of satisfaction within health-care organizations for any of these systems is very low, and they are simply waiting to be replaced. The good news is that new and some established enterprises outside the health-care system are accelerating innovation and developing solutions that will make the existing systems more usable and extend value on

36

the back end. For the existing systems, innovative companies are developing user-friendly interfaces that make it easier for physicians, nurses, and patients to enter information. On the back end, IBM, using Watson, and a host of start-ups are developing new solutions that leverage the power of artificial intelligence, reinforcement learning, and data science to better inform care paths and, if necessary, treatment decisions. They will become, sooner rather than later, an indispensable tool to the best physicians.

The most impactful change will come from smart, self-diagnosing technology. It promises to unlock unprecedented autonomy, control, and knowledge historically constrained by outdated technology and the existing physician practice model. These innovations afford health consumers real-time, personalized information and the ability to provide a level of self-service as well as new knowledge to intelligently manage their chronic conditions on their own. This new model promises to provide people fighting chronic conditions with the personalized experience they need and desire, with a solution that can be distributed across populations cost effectively and efficiently.

As costs have moved from acute to chronic conditions, the need for a new model is clear. Fortunately, circumstances now exist for creating such a model. That said, the key stakeholders in the industry have been slow to develop and adopt new innovations. Recognizing the opportunity, venture-capital firms are aggressively funding technology companies to develop solutions across health care, but particularly for people with chronic conditions. And having largely run out of money to continue to fund the double-digit increases of health-care expenses over the last 10 years, many of the country's largest self-insured employers are taking charge. One good example is the recent press release from Amazon, JPMorgan Chase, and Berkshire Hathaway, announcing that they will set up their own new nonprofit company to address the costs and quality of health care, a shot at payers and PBMs who traditionally were supposed to play that role but have been accused of only focusing on their own bottom lines. And many employers are much more open to trying new services to rein in costs. They are driving change to better assist their employees dealing with any number of chronic health conditions by looking outside the traditional avenues of the health-care system. They are beginning to invest in more effective solutions and, in doing so, reap the benefit of reducing costs while improving the health and happiness of their employees. Payers, seeing their customers getting out in front of them, are understanding the need to adopt innovations to improve care and, at the same time, reduce spending. Pharmacy benefit managers (PBMs)

> **"Many of the country's largest self-insured employers are taking charge."**

38

are also seeing the need to discover a new role focused as equally on improving care as on the bottom line. Interestingly, the most progressive and innovative payers and PBMs have accepted the need to reinvent themselves and are partnering with innovative smaller firms, blending the size and scale they enjoy

> **"The ACA has forever altered the makeup and dynamic of the health-care system."**

with the innovation they require, which is most often found in the smaller companies. And the best among them, like Cambia Health Solutions, no longer consider themselves payers at all. Mark Ganz, CEO of Cambia, says, "Our goal is no longer to function as a payer in the traditional sense. We want to embrace a new role for our customers, one focused on establishing relationships and creating value for the people we serve by helping them navigate to the best care that they and their families deem to be of highest value." To keep their eyes on innovation, payers and provider systems are setting up their own investment arms, investing directly, and in some cases, even starting new companies to ensure they are competitive and consumer focused in the future. For example, Cambia, mentioned above, has both partnered with Livongo to work together to create new products and, through their Echo Ventures venture-capital arm, invested in the company.

The ACA has forever altered the makeup and dynamic

of the health-care system. Unbeknownst to almost everyone involved and affected by its early passage, the most important impact may well have been understanding the impact health consumers could have when given the opportunity or forced to take responsibility for managing their own health. The aftermath of this landmark legislation, whether by plan or happenstance, has marshalled a new environment that forces health consumers to accept more accountability than ever before. This evolution now opens the door to address the chronic-condition epidemic cost effectively and sustainably.

• • •

Chapter Summary

- "The turbulence created by the ACA has led to the emergence of a new and increasingly powerful player in the health-care equation: the informed, connected health consumer."

- "The emergence of this new kind of health consumer has led to a watershed moment that will increasingly call into question why the system cannot provide the same information and service experience as today's most forward-thinking and innovative enterprises—such as

Amazon, Uber, Apple, and less well-known companies like Zeel, which locates massage therapists and sends them to your home on demand, and TalkSpace, which provides mental health support—who combine digital smarts with services in ways that increase satisfaction, demand, and a willingness to pay!"

- "The most impactful change will come from smart, self-diagnosing technology. It promises to unlock unprecedented autonomy, control, and knowledge historically constrained by outdated technology and the existing physician practice model. These innovations afford health consumers real-time, personalized information and the ability to provide a level of self-service as well as new knowledge to intelligently manage their chronic conditions on their own."

42

PART II:

THE NEW ORDER

CHAPTER 3:
TAKING A NEW APPROACH TO CHRONIC CONDITIONS

" *Every day the world turns upside down on someone who thought they were sitting on top of it.*"

:: Unknown

The future of managing chronic conditions rests in shifting the responsibility from the health-care "system" to informed, connected health consumers who are best positioned to make the greatest difference in their own health. This transition will be a difficult shift for many key participants in the health-care system. Their worlds will turn upside down as these newly informed and demanding consumers take charge. The key to making this shift successful centers on the process of *empowerment*—in other words, equipping those affected by chronic conditions with the tools and knowledge they need in order to take full ownership of their health, which we believe will produce far better and more sustainable clinical and financial results than traditional disease management programs.

Empowerment is a process, not an event, and it begins with the recognition that sustainable health improvement comes from the inside, not from the outside. We can't improve health by forcing it upon those with chronic conditions, but rather, we must enable them to opt in on their terms. Much of the underlying source of chronic conditions remains the lifestyle behaviors deeply ingrained in human psychology and the subsequent behaviors that require a personal commitment and desire to change. No one wants to suffer more from a chronic condition. At the same time, few people want to be told how to live, especially when that advice makes the process of staying healthy more difficult and burdensome. At

"No one wants to suffer more from a chronic condition."

present, the health-care system takes an outside-in approach toward "engaging" people in improving their health. While the best health-care organizations are redesigning their patient-care experience to accommodate patients, they are still ignoring the larger problem of redesigning how people spend their time outside the health-care system, which turns out to be most of their time (99 percent of it). By using technology to "empower" people, which implies action, rather than "engage" people, which implies participation, it becomes much easier to improve health on the individual's terms, creating the conditions for positive, sustainable behavior change. Remember, no one needed to engage you to use Google, Uber, Airbnb, or a host of our other favorite, value-adding applications.

Technology is the fundamental driver that makes the

45

empowerment model possible. Without it, the formula simply cannot work to facilitate successful behavior change at scale. To truly empower health consumers, the health-care system must embrace proven innovations from other industries that combine real-time information and data science to systematically generate greater value for everyone involved. No longer can the health-care system constrain information

"The formula simply cannot work to facilitate successful behavior change at scale."

to time, location, and price, or resist the innovations present in today's best-in-class categories, such as those pioneered by Amazon, Apple, and ride-sharing companies like Lyft, which seamlessly combine a digital experience with a service. Rather, the health-care system must empower everyone in the health-care equation with new knowledge to predict, prescribe, and prevent or at least delay the chronic-condition epidemic that we face. That thought can be challenging at best and even scary if your business model is based on people showing up for care. It means asking hospitals to engage in activities that ensure fewer of the same people come to them for treatment, which means less business unless they can grow their base. It's as if theaters told customers that they could also watch movies at home using Netflix. While theaters didn't make that suggestion, consumers have increasingly figured it out on their own. The result is that the largest film production companies today are Netflix and Amazon.

Consider several examples of innovations that have transformed the consumer experience. The first introduction of this capability, somewhat before its time, may have been OnStar, a driver-assistance technology introduced nearly two decades ago that provided drivers with 24/7 support in the case of a car crash. In its infancy, OnStar combined sensors, wireless technology, and the use of global positioning satellite technology (GPS) to track when and where drivers had an accident; connected them with real-time, in-person, remote support; and coordinated emergency response as necessary. The solution solved a critical problem for drivers, who in a crash previously remained at the mercy of whoever had witnessed it and could provide assistance, and in cases where no one was around, suffered the consequences. With OnStar, drivers now feel more secure and protected—whenever and wherever they experience a crash, even if they are unconscious. The value of the innovation did not rest in the technology itself but in the experience that it created. The

> "The value of the innovation did not rest in the technology itself but in the experience that it created."

process of getting from A to B did not change, only the degree of fear and anxiety people would experience after a crash.

CHAPTER 3: TAKING A NEW APPROACH TO CHRONIC CONDITIONS

OnStar never imposed itself on drivers by becoming ever-present; it only appeared at the exact moment drivers needed and wanted to use it. OnStar has saved many lives over the years and has become more understood and appreciated over time. However, the fundamental difference between OnStar and the kind of change we need in health care today is that OnStar didn't challenge the people who sold cars, nor did it disrupt their fundamental business model. It was an add-on.

Uptake, brilliantly founded by my friend Brad Keywell, is a company providing analytics solutions to industrial companies, and it provides another example, even closer to home. The Chicago-based enterprise takes OnStar's model of responsive service to the next level, using sensors and data science and analytics to provide predictive solutions to organizations operating equipment around the world. It is, in essence, keeping equipment "healthy" and "operating at 100 percent efficiency" by using data from sensors on the equipment to anticipate (predict) when checkups and service visits are needed. And then it sends technicians out (think prescribing a house call) rather than waiting for the equipment to fail and need to be serviced. All this to prevent a costly breakdown. For instance, Uptake helps construction companies keep equipment working. For large infrastructure projects, cranes serve as critical assets that can dramatically impact the cost and schedule. A crane that malfunctions or is out of service can halt an entire project, resulting in delays that may span days or weeks and cost millions of dollars. To prevent downtime, Uptake embeds sensors in Caterpillar construction equipment to monitor and diagnose the health of cranes in real time. Tracking this equipment around the globe, the company accumulates vast amounts of data and uses analytics to understand patterns that result in downtime

> **"The company accumulates vast amounts of data and uses analytics to understand patterns that result in downtime and predict how and when to intervene."**

and predict how and when to intervene. Before a crane breaks down, the company sends mechanics on-site to make the necessary repairs, replacements, or updates to equipment that to the naked eye, may seem like it is running perfectly fine. Uptake takes the OnStar model a step further by predicting, prescribing (service), and thereby preventing interruptions. It eliminates scheduled service that may or may not be needed and replaces it with real-life prevention and proactive repairs to safeguard against costly downtime. Interestingly, in an industry where price had become the only differentiator, Uptake's technology returned Caterpillar's competitive advantage and pricing stability. Uptime—also known as staying on schedule—is the most important metric to someone building a skyscraper.

Imagine if we could combine the preventive aspects of

49

Uptake with the emergency interventions of OnStar and treat people—our most important asset—with that kind of care! *Predicting* who needs to visit their physician and who can skip their quarterly checkup; *prescribing* drug therapies based on individuals' specific indications, and as important, nutrition and exercise regimens, and other healthy interventions; and *preventing* the downtime (the condition) from ever happening in the

> **"'Technology, perfectly applied, is indistinguishable from magic.'"**

first place. When it does happen, imagine being there at the exact moment someone needs help but only when someone really needs assistance in managing their health issues. We've all had a medical situation where we wished we had a doctor present or could talk with one in the moment. If the phone rang at just that moment, we would call it perfect timing, as many of our members at Livongo say when our certified diabetes educators call. Arthur C. Clarke said, "Technology, perfectly applied, is indistinguishable from magic." In other words, if we could create a perfect experience using technology, that would be magical. That's our future, but we must lean into it, or as I like to say, *lead* into it.

In the health-care system, we need to apply similar innovations to provide the best and most effective experience for people with chronic conditions. And remember, it's all about the experience, not the technology. Imagine the sense of control, protection, relief, and satisfaction health consumers would feel with similar empowerment to manage their chronic conditions. Instead of living in the constant worries of a chronic condition, they could immediately and easily gain access to the

"The job of the health system is to give you that control back."

information and support they need and desire, the kind of power that would enable them to almost forget about their condition, at least temporarily, and begin to focus on living. Remember, a chronic condition always takes something away, and in most cases, it's control over some aspect of the individual's life. The job of the health system is to give you that control back. What's interesting and why this new approach is so different than traditional health care is that control may be as simple as information, measurement, awareness, or a connection to a community of like-minded people sharing a similar experience, like managing a chronic condition. While the technology does have a cost, most of what it delivers can actually be free and can have a significant impact.

Technology now provides the opportunity to manage chronic conditions effectively in everyday life, but creating the conditions for true behavior change depends on three fundamental factors:

51

(1) How we empower health consumers with information
(2) How we build and provide access to a caring community of people
(3) How we provide real-time, context-aware care

It all begins with making information available to people. In the past, we seemed to think—like the travel industry thought we couldn't book our own travel—that patients couldn't manage health-care information. But increasingly, websites like WebMD, which attracts more than 183 million searches on average each month, and many others have demonstrated that not only can patients research and self-diagnose, but the internet is the first place they look.[10] We are in the early stages of the development of this resource. Today, the internet includes all kinds of information with few tools for patients to assess what's real and relevant, and what isn't. To make the internet more effective, we need to make the information personalized, simple, actionable, and context aware. For example, if your phone rings and someone says they will arrive in 15 minutes to fix your tire, you're not happy to receive that call . . . unless you have a flat tire. Then you often respond, "Perfect

> "It all begins with making information available to people."

[10] Shaheen Kanthawala, Amber Vermeesch, Barbara Given, and Jina Huh, "Answers to Health Questions: Internet Search Results Versus Online Health Community Responses," *Journal of Medical Internet Research*, 18, no. 4, April 2016, DOI:10.2196/jmir.5369

timing," or, "What a coincidence you called." But imagine that it wasn't a coincidence. Imagine that your tire contained a sensor that alerted the closest tire repair shop with the lowest cost and highest quality that your tire needed to be fixed, and then the repair shop sent out a mobile van—all without you knowing it. Magic! We need to use technology to create that same magic moment by understanding the *body's vital narrative*—the unique story the body tells each of us and the signals it gives us—and then, through science, what we should do to improve it.

Second, we must build a caring community to help provide responsive care to people with chronic conditions when they need it. People can become part of the care network, but only when they are informed about the health needs of an individual. This means empowering the caring community—which includes anyone who can help—with information to know when and how to support those in need. Family members, friends, coworkers, roommates, and others closest to those with chronic conditions should understand when and how to offer support. Everyone can benefit from a growing pool of information about the factors that lead to better or worse outcomes, information that, combined with data science, can identify predictive, prescriptive, and preventative treatments based on individual characteristics.

Information and the caring community only work if they are offered in real time, in context, and they expand care

53

beyond physicians and hospitals. Real time calls for responding to the needs of the individual at the perfect moment when they need assistance. In context—i.e., being context aware—entails providing solutions that fit the current situation and provide the most impactful health benefits. And expanding care means providing whatever people need to stay healthy on their terms, whether it's information, someone to speak with, a community to consult with, people nearby to provide support and assistance, or encouragement from family, friends, and connections. It also means knowing when you need a doctor and when you don't. Care, in this sense, requires a fundamentally new definition with the informed, connected health consumer at the center. We must use technology to provide real-time, context-aware care to ensure health consumers receive the support they need when they need it and prevent unnecessary and expensive trips to the emergency room or the hospital. All three factors remain essential to creating the conditions that empower people to manage their chronic condition cost effectively and sustainably at the population level. Simply stated, better health, happier people, at lower costs—and less traditional health care!

Empowerment leads to better, more sustainable outcomes for everyone involved, including physicians, who today are not seeing the right patients and often not getting rewarded properly, either economically or in job satisfaction. However, people have to want to become healthier, and we believe they do, but only if we can make it easier and more rewarding for them to stay healthy. If behavior change represents the solution to chronic conditions, then one of the most important indicators of improved health is whether people with chronic conditions will embrace the empowerment model. The more satisfied they feel, the more likely they will continue to foster and reinforce healthier lifestyle changes. The better they feel, the more positive their clinical results and the greater the cost savings. Nearly 90 percent of people with chronic conditions report being satisfied with the empowerment model,[11] while 75 percent also feel more confident about their conditions.[12] Both figures translate into high rates of adherence, with 80 percent of consumers using real-time feedback to engage in healthier behaviors.[13] Compared with traditional disease management programs, this represents over a 60 percent improvement.[14] Combining these results with clinical and financial outcomes demonstrates the overall value of the empowerment model. For large, self-insured employers, results show that empowerment produces significant clinical benefits in populations with diabetes and cardiovascular disease.[15] For diabetes, empowerment results in a reduction in the likelihood of having an out-of-range blood glucose reading[16]—an event that poses a significant risk for complications[17]—and also results in a reduction in

55

---

[11] *Livongo Clinical and Financial Outcomes Report.* Mountain View: Livongo Health, June 2016. Accessed August 14, 2017. https://www.livongo.com/docs/pdf/Livongo%20Clinical%20and%20Financial%20Outcomes%20Report.pdf

[12] "Livongo Net Promoter Score from Member Satisfaction Survey." Livongo Health, September 2016.

[13] ibid

[14] *World Health Organization: Adherence to long-term therapies. Evidence for action.* Geneva: World Health Organization; 2003.

[15] Source: Livongo client biometric screening. Difference-in-difference method—i.e., Livongo pre-post versus non-Livongo over same time.

[16] Janelle Downing, Jenna Bollyky, Jennifer Schneider. "Use of a Connected Glucose Meter and Certified Diabetes Educator Coaching to Decrease the Likelihood of Abnormal Blood Glucose Excursions: The Livongo for Diabetes Program." *Journal of Medical Internet Research* 19, no.7 (July 2017), Accessed August 14, 2017. DOI: 10.2196/jmir.6659

[17] Results from Livongo client biometric screening show an average reduction of 17 percent in the likelihood of having an out-of-range blood glucose reading.

A1C.[18] Interestingly, diabetes is also an umbrella disease. If someone feels bad because their blood sugar is very high, they are less likely to take their medications for other conditions or exercise. They also experience depression at higher rates. If we can empower health-care consumers to control their diabetes, other conditions improve as well. Studies show better glycemic control (control over blood sugar) improves hypertension, dyslipidemia (elevated blood cholesterol), obesity, and depression.[19] For populations with cardiovascular disease, results indicate that the empowerment model reduces total cholesterol and triglycerides significantly.[20] The improvement in clinical results, combined with a more cost-effective model, leads to significant savings. A number of recent studies have shown that large, self-insured employers are able to save between $75 and $100 per participating member per month compared with similar populations not participating in the programs.

The opportunity now exists to create the conditions that truly change behavior sustainably and across populations. The health-care system and its participants, including physicians, need to begin to recognize the need to shift the responsibility of managing chronic conditions to the people impacted by them, and technology now exists that makes this shift not

56

---

[18] Results from Livongo client biometric screening show an average reduction of nearly 1 percent in HbA1c over 270 days, from 7.7 to 6.9 percent.

[19] Mary Ann Banjeri, and Jeffrey D. Dunn, "Impact of Glycemic Control on Healthcare Resource Utilization and Costs of Type 2 Diabetes: Current and Future Pharmacologic Approaches to Improving Outcomes," *American Health & Drug Benefits*, September 2013, https://www.ncbi.nlm.nih.gov/pmc/articles/PMC4031727/

[20] Results from Livongo client biometric screening show an average reduction of total cholesterol by 37 percent and triglycerides by 8.3 percent.

only possible but valuable to the person with the condition. What remains is the need to accelerate the shift underway and commit to truly empowering health consumers to improve their health on their own terms.

• • •

Chapter Summary

- "The future of managing chronic conditions rests in shifting the responsibility from the health-care 'system' to informed, connected health consumers who are best positioned to make the greatest difference in their own health."

- "By using technology to 'empower' people, which implies action, rather than 'engage' people, which implies participation, it becomes much easier to improve health on the individual's terms, creating the conditions for positive, sustainable behavior change."

- "Rather, the health-care system must empower everyone in the health-care equation with new knowledge to predict, prescribe, and prevent or at least delay the chronic-condition epidemic that we face."

58

PART III:

EMPOWERING THE NEW HEALTH CONSUMER

Chapter 4:
Empowering the Informed Connected Health Consumer with Information

❝ *The future is already here; it's just not evenly distributed."*

:: William Gibson

Several years ago, I published an article in *Forbes* on why the health-care system's "engagement" approach—getting the patient more actively involved in their own health care—doesn't work. While the article drew instant interest, some people disagreed with it. They thought I argued that people should not become more engaged in their health, which wasn't the point. My thesis was based on our research at Livongo, from people managing their own chronic conditions—people who told us they wanted freedom from the conditions that affected them, to spend more time living their lives and less time focused on their conditions. They wanted the power to live healthier while also making the task of getting there less burdensome and time consuming. *They wanted to be less engaged and more empowered.* That was the point. The people we interviewed wanted to use technology to shoulder the burden of living with a chronic condition. They cited tools they used frequently in other aspects of their lives—the Amazons,

Facebooks, and Apples of the world—and wondered why similar solutions couldn't enable them to more effectively manage their hypertension, diabetes, weight issues, or mental health issues, and spend less time.

Simply stated, the health-care consumers wanted to be less engaged with their disease. In my article, I wasn't arguing that people should become less engaged in their health but rather that they wanted to be more empowered to manage their health on their terms and not someone else's.

Our greatest chance of solving the chronic-condition epidemic in this country and across the world requires us to look to the last place we might imagine: the person who is living with chronic disease on a daily basis. This calls for putting our faith in those with the greatest power to make a difference. And it starts by recognizing that people with chronic conditions can and should make most of their health decisions. To do so requires us to empower them with the information and tools to make the right decisions on their terms. Surprisingly, or maybe not, we do know what's best for us and what will work best for our health! Remember, health decisions are not made in a silo but in context of a million other family, income, work, and personal considerations. We also need to understand that while

> "Simply stated, the health-care consumers wanted to be less engaged with their disease."

technology can help enable this transition of power, it is not the panacea. The value comes from the experience it allows us to create. To truly empower informed, connected health consumers, we must enable them to design and create the experience most appropriate for them and make it personal, context sensitive, and real time. This requires empowering them with information to make more intelligent decisions, while ensuring new knowledge remains connected to their psychological and physiological needs. Only then can we create the conditions for sustainable behavior change and a new environment that empowers people to stay healthy, happy, and free from more invasive and expensive medical interventions—and have the ability to scale the same model across broader populations.

Health care is an information business, and the sooner we accept that the better. We are moving away from the traditional, provider-centric model to one built around consumers and their health awareness. Today, we talk about health care. But the reality is that there are two very different sectors—health care and health (and fitness)—and both are coming together. The real solution lies in between both. The traditional health-care system is centered on "fixing" problems that patients have, and

"Health care is an information business, and the sooner we accept that the better."

the health (and fitness) industry is focused on providing people with tools such as apps, devices, and experiences to proactively address health. While the health-care industry remains slow to adopt new technology and innovations, the health industry continues to innovate and introduce

> "The health industry continues to innovate and introduce new solutions at a blistering pace."

new solutions at a blistering pace. Fitbit is an exceptional example of the type of innovation and connected devices that can empower the informed, connected health consumer. They provide people with new knowledge about their health to encourage them to embrace healthier habits. Fitbit draws on psychology to motivate people to adopt better behaviors, using the simple science of goal setting to motivate consumers to do more than yesterday's achievements. Despite these advancements, health and fitness tools still primarily focus on healthy and health-conscious people, or as some would call them, the "worried well." While they do increase awareness (and are a step in the right direction), they remain inadequate to address the challenges of chronic conditions. They are designed for people who have yet to feel the true weight of living with a chronic condition. People with chronic conditions require far more—from the type of information they receive to the experience they demand—to "engage," act,

63

and stay healthy. While Fitbit users generally want to spend more time, energy, and attention on their health, people with chronic conditions want to spend less time, but so far, solutions continue to ignore this discrepancy and leave people with chronic conditions to manage their health on their own without access to good information or support. Fitbit's most recently announced $6 million investment in Sano, a Silicon Valley-based startup that is developing a minimally invasive continuous blood glucose monitor, is a step in the right direction, bridging the gap between health and health care. It represents one of many partnerships forming between the two sectors, combining wearable devices with sensors to track blood glucose in real time.[21]

While we can talk about health care and health fitness, I believe a third segment is emerging. This space focuses on providing people with chronic conditions the information and support they need to live beyond the four walls of the hospital or their doctor's office. Sensors that enable self-monitoring and sharing technology now provide people with the ability to better understand their health status in real time, removing the gray area between lifestyle behaviors and health that traditionally leaves people unaware and unmotivated to make better decisions. These tools also provide insights about better behaviors and capitalize on the opportunity to empower people with new knowledge that allows them to actively engage

[21] "Fitbit invests $6M in glucose monitoring startup Sano," *MobiHealthNews*, January 08, 2018, http://www.mobihealthnews.com/content/fitbit-invests-6m-glucose-monitoring-startup-sano

in their own care. These new technologies can provide real-time metrics, personalized analysis, and recommendations at the "perfect" moments when people need, want, and are ready to absorb information from which they can truly benefit. They can also suggest when people need additional help managing their condition.

Despite advancements made in mobile, cellular, and remote patient monitoring technology, most tools remain inadequate to truly empower people. Rather than information, they provide data. The new generation of tools needs to provide not just metrics but insights, suggestions, and actions for people with chronic conditions to address their needs in a way that creates an experience that motivates them to change their behaviors sustainably.

65

One example, near and dear to my heart, comes from the diabetes space. Traditional glucose meters (devices used to measure blood sugar) simply provide a number with no guidance, trending, or valuable insights. They fail to meet the same standards as the best-in-class solutions proven in other industries, providing insufficient information to build awareness, interest, and motivation. Dr. William Polonsky, president of the Behavioral Diabetes

"The new generation of tools needs to provide not just metrics but insights, suggestions, and actions."

Institute and a leading expert on behavioral issues for people with diabetes, explains the challenge perfectly: "The problem with blood glucose meters is, they don't tell us what our numbers mean or what we're supposed to do with them. They only tell us that our numbers are high or low. Without better information, many of us see our numbers as a statement of whether we've been good or bad. We feel ashamed, and over time, our natural inclination is to avoid the numbers altogether."

Most of these solutions cannot personalize information to create the conditions for the best outcomes, not to mention leverage psychology to drive people to change. They also do not ease the burden of living with a chronic condition and instead require manual tasks that technology can easily automate. This causes frustration and fatigue that ultimately leads to nonadherence. Many tools also miss the mark in capturing the appropriate context in which people find themselves. They fail to provide learning at the moment when people are actively engaged in their health. Today's solutions neglect the fundamental principles needed to empower people to achieve their best health and feel motivated and energized in the process—principles that are common in

> "Many tools also miss the mark in capturing the appropriate context in which people find themselves."

practically every other industry. While many tools increase access to data, few turn that data into usable information or consider the broader experiences and context

> **"People will gain real insight into their *body's vital narrative* whenever and wherever they want."**

that drive or detract people from staying healthy.

Newer, more sophisticated solutions are emerging that promise to transform how people experience and manage their chronic conditions. Driven by smart devices, connectivity to the cloud, and deep data science, paired with the behavioral understanding Dr. Polonsky mentions, these new solutions will create the conditions for optimal health by providing information that produces the best outcome for each individual and experiences people appreciate and want to continue. For the first time, people will gain real insight into their *body's vital narrative* whenever and wherever they want, as well as insights uniquely tailored to their needs delivered at just the right time. These new solutions leverage the four principles common to successful solutions in other industries. To empower the consumer, new solutions and the information they provide must be personalized, context aware, simple, and actionable. Early evidence shows that solutions with these characteristics will be effective in improving health and motivation. In fact, research shows that 80 percent of people

67

actively use information from these devices to engage in healthier behaviors. Simply put, this new generation of devices that enable information represents the future of managing the health of populations through a more personalized and consumer-driven approach to care.

Personalize the Process to Drive Meaning, Value, and Better Outcomes

A personalized approach to care starts by recognizing that chronic conditions are as unique and nuanced as the people affected by them. Type 2 Diabetes affects everyone differently, so to treat the condition rather than the person means to ignore the psychological and physiological factors that continue to drive behaviors we may want to change. A far better approach recognizes the need to treat the individual first and the condition second, because when it comes to chronic conditions, the individual often serves as the cause of and solution to the problem.

This personalized approach to care represents the only viable and sustainable solution to managing the health of populations. We can no longer focus on perfecting costly treatments while neglecting the people ultimately affected by them. Instead, we must focus on how to empower people with information tailored to their needs to get them actively involved rather than passively responsive. Information serves as the most cost-effective solution in the fight against chronic conditions, and while it remains scarce in today's health-care model, technology can deliver critical information in real time, at just the right time, to leverage the traditionally unharnessed power of those affected. The more we personalize information, the more people embrace it and the more effective it becomes.

Personalized information creates the conditions for better outcomes by making the process meaningful to recipients and providing new knowledge that reflects their exact needs. The more we customize information to the individual, the more he or she invariably perceives value and meaning in it. This remains true of any context, but particularly health. If I call and tell you to visit your doctor twice a year, then you may or may not listen to my advice. But if I call and say that your lab results are ready and the doctor would like to see you, you can't book an appointment fast enough. This is a consistent behavior for everyone. Why? Because the message becomes personal instead of general. The more we supply people with new knowledge that reflects their exact condition and experience, the more likely they will

> **"The more we customize information to the individual, the more he or she invariably perceives value and meaning in it."**

take actions that lead to better health. Today, we are starting to understand the individual characteristics and behaviors that make chronic conditions unique, such as the differences in how people absorb insulin if they exercise regularly or how men and women react to different medications. In the past, we ignored these differences, instead treating the condition rather than the health consumer. Now, we can begin to address the factors that result in different outcomes and choose only the best actions for each individual to achieve better or optimal health.

How do we personalize information to drive meaning and optimal outcomes? By looking at today's proven innovations to understand how they empower consumers with information and experiences tailored uniquely to them. Facebook doesn't provide a general experience for the people who use it, nor does Amazon. The millions of consumers shopping on Amazon each day expect an experience tailored to their needs and behaviors. They expect to be welcomed with instant access to sections titled "Recommended for you" or "You may also be interested in," sections listing products curated specifically for them based on past purchases and behaviors. They expect an experience that they find meaningful and that drives greater efficiency, but also effectiveness—i.e., introducing them to new products and

"They expect an experience that they find meaningful and that drives greater efficiency, but also effectiveness."

knowledge that can alter their everyday lives. Imagine a similar model applied in the management of chronic conditions—one that empowers those affected with information to create a better experience, both by capitalizing on what consumers value and find meaningful, and by exposing them to new knowledge that leads to better outcomes. Just as consumers on Amazon receive recommendations based on items they searched and bought previously, imagine people with chronic conditions receiving personalized recommendations that account for their characteristics—such as gender, ethnicity, age, diet restrictions, etc.—as well as their behaviors: sleep patterns, exercise habits, medications, etc. And while we're speaking largely of clinical information, this is an opportunity to build a database of what actually works. While each response provides personalized information, we can also begin to learn from other people with similar characteristics, habits, and psychological makeup, and share that information in an appropriate way. To increase their likelihood of adhering to these recommendations, we should call out the optimal benefits the behavior has produced for people with similar characteristics. For the first time, we can use data science and the power of the crowd. But we must have data. Currently, in diabetes, that data resides in millions of unconnected meters, which makes it of no use to anyone. In hypertension, to the extent that people are checking their blood pressure at home, which is the best place to check it, that data is almost

71

never shared. In a model of connected care, however, that data becomes information that can be shared across entire populations. People with diabetes and hypertension receive personalized recommendations for managing their conditions that account for their physiological needs and behavioral patterns. Greater personalization produces better results, and with better results, people feel more empowered and compelled to remain engaged and motivated in the pursuit of better health.

This is the kind of community—a connected, valuable community—that we can create for people living with chronic conditions. While each response is personalized, imagine the value of sharing recommendations of what other people did and found beneficial in managing their chronic condition—and doing so in an appropriate way that people actually find valuable. In the example of Amazon, imagine informed, connected health consumers gaining access to information marked "Recommended for people like you in this context." The value not only comes from the knowledge that information is personalized but is connected to entire populations contributing to and benefiting from the network.

Increase Context Awareness to Add Relevance and Drive Better Value

Solutions only work in a certain context. Even personalized information is not valuable in the wrong setting or at the wrong time. For example, a low blood sugar reading requires a different solution than a normal or high reading, just as a series of low readings calls for a different solution than a single occurrence. Context-aware information takes personalization a step further by recognizing that health remains an ever-evolving state. It extends personalized care to account for the needs of the present as opposed to the past or the future. Great care takes place in the present—in real time. Delivering the right information at the right time is critical to the success of the new, emerging health-care model, which revolves around informed, connected consumers—not "patients" in the traditional sense of the word.

For example, we believe that 85 percent of seizures caused by low blood sugar in people with Type 1 Diabetes could be prevented. Most show early warning signs that if identified and understood, and then appropriately treated, could not only prevent the seizure but would reduce the trauma, risk, and cost normally associated with such events. Seizures occur

73

"Think about the risks when people with critically low blood sugar decide to drive or operate machinery."

when blood sugar runs too low and your body reacts by shutting down nonessential systems—like walking and talking—to protect your heart and brain, to keep you alive. The first stage may be dizziness or impacted decision making and then fainting. Think about the risks when people with critically low blood sugar decide to drive or operate machinery. They may not realize the life-threatening danger, should they experience a seizure. But imagine the value of information delivered in real time that alerts them how their body is trending, notifies others so they can help, and reminds them of what to do if they are not thinking clearly. Think about predicting, prescribing, and preventing. If we notice a trend of very low blood sugars, we can actively intervene. Imagine the change we can achieve—in both human and financial terms. Context-aware information is not only necessary but critical to keeping people healthy and protected.

How can we make information more context aware? Like personalization, the answer centers on learning from and leveraging many of the proven innovations found in other industries that make context-aware knowledge possible. In chapter three, we explored the examples of OnStar and Uptake to illustrate the value of using technology and remote sensing to provide responsive service tailored to a unique problem of consumers as well as developing solutions that predict and prevent problems before they occur. We can apply the same model to chronic conditions. For diabetes specifically, we can empower people with information to better manage their blood sugar

"We can empower people with information to better manage their blood sugar to normal levels."

to normal levels as well as provide them with new knowledge that identifies patterns of health. For example, a low blood sugar reading might trigger a recommendation to drink three ounces of juice and check blood sugar again in 30 minutes—all depending on the person and his or her needs at the current moment. If it was before lunch, it would be treated very differently than after lunch. Context means everything. Similarly, a person with a high blood sugar reading would receive instructions to drink more water instead of juice, walk for a specified period, and recheck their blood glucose. If a person with diabetes experiences a series of low blood sugar readings after several days, they may receive information to consult with their physician about the amount of insulin they are using to avoid taking too much, or it may tell them to eat more carbs before bed to raise their blood sugar slowly. It would also warn the person of his or her increased risk of a seizure, providing recommendations to remain healthy and safe. OnStar uses sensors to alert you after a crash and provides the current status of your car, but to continue the analogy, we're more interested in the health of the passenger and preventing the crash in the first place. The next stage is providing health consumers with smart, connected, information-enabled devices that track their *body's vital narrative* and intervene with information at the perfect moment when people need it—before the crash. And like Uptake, health consumers need the power of the cloud and data science to understand their *body's vital narrative* and analyze patterns to predict, prescribe, and prevent bad health outcomes.

Today, we're continuing to learn, as health consumers, about our bodies so we can understand what we need to feel and perform at our best. Tomorrow, that may not be the case. While at present, we rely on the inaccurate science of intuition to guess what we need to feel well—a cup of coffee in the morning, a walk during lunch, a good book before bed—in the future, we will rely on science to figure out exactly what our bodies need to function at peak performance all the time.

Simplify the Process of Staying Healthy

Part of restoring control to the people affected by chronic conditions entails simplifying the process of staying healthy. The simpler we make it to be and stay healthy, the more likely people will behave in ways that improve their overall health. Every step we automate and simplify makes it more likely that someone will make a good decision rather than a less healthy one.

Technology handles the tasks we don't like and don't always perform well. People don't like balancing their checkbook and technology has provided a solution for that and more. People with diabetes don't like manually recording their test results after each blood glucose reading, storing them, and bringing them to their physician on quarterly visits, not to mention remembering to order and pay for more test strips, which can be very expensive. They perceive these tasks as unnecessary, given their knowledge of solutions capable of saving them time and effort—innovations ever-present in other aspects of their lives. No one manually records and tracks their finances—technology automates our banking. Asking people to perform tasks that technology can complete more proficiently only discourages and disengages them from activities that make a difference in their health.

People want the experience of managing a chronic condition to reflect the ease and automation of a pacemaker. Pacemakers—surgically implanted devices that regulate abnormal heartbeats continuously and automatically— 77 continue to save, prolong, and improve lives with minimal effort from the people who wear them. The beauty of this technology is what it allows people to forget. Outside of the initial

> **"The beauty of this technology is what it allows people to forget."**

surgery, many people practically forget the device is inside their body; meanwhile, it keeps them alive and their heart working normally without disrupting everyday living. People affected by chronic conditions want similar innovations that enable them to live normally. They want the process to become easier and less burdensome, not to mention less isolating. The more seamless the process, the more engaged people feel in promoting healthier behaviors. Conversely, the more intrusive the process, the more it reminds people of their condition and the more they avoid its management altogether.

One afternoon, I walked downstairs and found my son playing a role-playing game (RPG). I wanted to join him, so I asked, "Where are the instructions?" "Dad," he responded, his voice taking the familiar tone of a teenager educating his parents, "nothing smart has instructions anymore." The notion that someone would need to read and learn to use a system or device before using it has become outdated. Today, we don't get out our phones and take a course on how to use them. No one taught people how to use Google, yet today, more than a billion people use it to better understand the world around them, including, increasingly, health-care patients, physicians, and professionals. Even if we get the spelling wrong on a search term, Google corrects it and almost always populates the results we intended to find. Google serves as a good example of a smart system that keeps learning about you based on your behaviors. Its PageRank algorithm, named after cofounder Larry Page, who designed it, displays

> "The notion that someone would need to read and learn to use a system or device before using it has become outdated."

results according to the most commonly selected choices that people make when using the search engine. The more people that select certain results, the higher Google displays them in search rankings. It learns about you and elevates your experience based on its understanding of your interests and behaviors. Amazon Prime serves as another good example. The system lists products you ordered previously to make it easier to make repeat purchases, recognizing that people often buy the same items for routine purchases such as toothpaste or detergent. Amazon Prime learns what you like and makes it incredibly easy to find. All smart systems learn, and this ability will improve in the future. We should expect similar intuitive interfaces that continue to become smarter over time from our health-care devices. How can we make the process of managing a chronic condition simpler? The answer is understanding where technology can help. It can manage information on a breadth and scope beyond the capabilities of any human. Technology, rather than people, should own the responsibility of collecting, tracking, storing, and disseminating health information, which for a person dealing with diabetes would include his or her blood glucose readings and a lot more, including the contextual information and what works and what doesn't. And because communication between people and their physicians remains notoriously cumbersome, technology should automate that too, sending only the most important results, insights, and answers to

79

physicians only when they need to see them rather than a huge amount of unstructured and often unusable data, which is common today. And when we translate data into information and insights, we make the process of staying healthy easier.

Traditional health care sends people to the physician when they become sick rather than empowering health consumers, who hold the greatest power to make a difference in their own health long before a physician visit or a hospital stay is necessary. At Livongo, we wanted to completely reinvent the experience for people with diabetes and began by listening to health consumers with chronic conditions, who perhaps not surprisingly told us that they wanted the process of staying healthy to become easier, not more difficult. We recognized the need to eliminate everything that health consumers didn't like and didn't want to do in the management of their health. That meant not just simplifying the process by attacking the consumer hassle map but also removing other barriers in the effort to improve health. The cost of test strips is a good example. The expensive test strips people buy each week cause some people, particularly those who are under-resourced, to check their blood glucose less frequently than they should— risking their overall health. The cost remains insignificant compared to a visit to the emergency room or a critical event. Rather than charge people for test strips, at Livongo, we thought a better approach was to make test strips free, recognizing that the downstream savings significantly outweigh the upfront costs. The more we can simplify the process of staying healthy, both from the standpoint of information and experience, the more effective we become at creating the conditions for people to engage in healthier living.

Make Real-Time Feedback Actionable

The next step is making information actionable. Having information and not knowing what to do with it or, worse, being told to take actions that are not practical, possible, or desirable leads to frustration and reduced compliance. In contrast, we know that actionable recommendations, tailored to the person and context, serve as the best approach to treating chronic conditions, as they address health incrementally and make the process manageable. No one wants information they need to remember or that needs to be translated by a medical

81

"The next step is making information actionable."

professional, but we know that everyone wants to be healthier and eliminate all of the challenges their chronic condition causes. Actionable information enables people to forget about their chronic condition until the appropriate moment when they need to address it and, when they do, manage it most effectively and efficiently. As Dr. Polonsky explains, we need to help people *interpret* their blood glucose numbers, not just record them. The more we provide interpretive support, the more we can help people feel and do better. This approach recognizes that the more we can guide people with direct, immediate, and actionable information, the less time they spend dwelling on concerns related to their conditions. Actionable information quiets the noise of a chronic condition by getting people to focus on the small behaviors that make the greatest impact on their overall health. The focus shifts from the condition itself to the task at hand. To crystalize everything down to a simple message—one that directs a specific, simple, achievable behavior in a certain time frame that leads to better health—enables people with chronic conditions to live beyond the shadow of their illness.

How can we make information actionable? By making it simple, immediate, and measurable. "Simple" means people can understand exactly what they need to do. "Immediate" refers to an action that people can perform in the moment and in their environment, not later.

> **"'Measurable' calls for providing people with a measurable outcome to gauge success."**

"Measurable" calls for providing people with a measurable outcome to gauge success. Combining these elements provides people with a clear objective that shifts their attention from dwelling on their conditions to taking proactive steps to address them. Recall the example of a context-aware message that tells people how to raise their blood sugar: "Drink three ounces of juice and check again in 30 minutes." When people check their blood sugar a second time and discover their blood glucose has moved in the right direction or returned to within range, their actions are reinforced and they feel rewarded in three ways: first, through the sense of accomplishment that comes with completing a task; second, by feeling healthier and better; and third, by knowing they can take charge of their condition and make a difference in their health. Together, the process produces satisfaction and confidence that build positive momentum in the journey toward better health. This is a good example of actionable information because it removes any doubt of what health consumers need to do now to start feeling better.

These four fundamental principles—making information personalized, context aware, simple, and actionable—produce experiences consumers want and need. Personalized information drives context-aware, simple, and actionable knowledge by accounting for the psychological and physiological factors that make each person unique. Context-aware information, on the other hand, enhances the other three principles by recognizing the current circumstances of individuals and the internal and external factors influencing their health in the moment. Making the process simple increases the value of personalized, context-aware, and actionable information by ensuring people remain engaged in the behaviors that improve their overall health. And actionable information translates personalized, context-aware, and simple knowledge into immediate behaviors that produce optimal results.

Technology does not serve as the ultimate answer to chronic conditions, but it enables the delivery of personalized, context-aware, simple, and actionable information. The more we can build on these principles to empower informed, connected health consumers with better experiences and solutions, the more we can begin to see improvements in health across populations of people. Information remains the least expensive and most available resource in the fight against chronic conditions. By carefully designing how we deliver it according to these four principles, we can create the conditions for enlisting the millions of people impacted by chronic conditions to manage and own more of the responsibility for staying healthy. Our success depends on how we use information to change a person's experience. Other industries are already consumer driven. Now it's time for health care to get on the information bandwagon. The better the experience, the more people embrace it and the more health we create for everyone.

• • •

Chapter Summary

- "Our greatest chance of solving the chronic-condition epidemic in this country and across the world requires us to look to the last place we might imagine: the person who is living with chronic disease on a daily basis."

- "Newer, more sophisticated solutions are emerging that promise to transform how people experience and manage their chronic conditions . . . These new solutions leverage the four principles common to successful solutions in other industries. To empower the consumer, new solutions and the information they provide must be personalized, context aware, simple, and actionable."

- "Information remains the least expensive and most available resource in the fight against chronic conditions. By carefully designing how we deliver it according to these four principles, we can create the conditions for enlisting the millions of people impacted by chronic conditions to manage and own more of the responsibility for staying healthy."

Chapter 5:
Building a Caring Community

" Invisible threads are the strongest ties."

:: Friedrich Nietzsche

At the corner of my desk sat a hot fudge sundae, a pleasant surprise after a busy afternoon. I almost didn't notice Chirine, my executive assistant, standing at the door.

"I brought you something," she said, smiling.

"Thanks. What did I do to deserve this?" I asked.

She had a small black monitoring device in her hand that I had left on her desk. It was the reader for the Dexcom G4 continuous glucose monitor (CGM) I was wearing. While I don't have diabetes, I often wear the latest devices to better understand the experience people with diabetes have when they are connected. The G4 is designed to continuously monitor blood sugar from the sensor attached to your stomach, which transmits the results in real time. Running between meetings, I had left the monitor on Chirine's desk.

"I noticed your blood sugar was low, and I know that low blood sugar can sometimes make people irritable. Since I'm meeting with you next, I wanted to ensure you were in a good mood!"

While we both laughed, it didn't take me long to realize the power of that moment and that it was truly a sign of things to come. Chirine, who is not a medical professional, knew more about what was happening in my own body at that moment than I did and took action to improve my mood, all without the slightest medical training. Imagine that at scale. Every day, we wake up and want to feel and perform our best, but we don't have the information, nor do we have the required actions to make that a reality. Both are required to achieve optimum health and performance. Now, imagine a world where we did. Imagine waking up and knowing exactly what you need to drink or eat, or the exercise you have to do to feel amazing. And we've all had that feeling of waking up and feeling rested and ready to take on the world. What if we could bottle that? And what if that magic elixir is already within reach? What if we could decode your *body's vital narrative* and know the secret to feeling amazing every day? Today, we are one step closer to that dream and we can, at least for blood sugar, know exactly where we are at a given point, where we're heading, and what to do to impact that.

There is a second point that is critically important. When others know you need support, they are happy to provide it. This is especially true when it comes to chronic conditions, but they need to know—they need the information. Imagine if you knew a good friend was feeling down and depressed. Would you call him or her? Most people would. When the

Livongo system provides a real-time text to the care network—family, friends, roommates, coworkers, and anyone else who needs and wants to know and is close by—that someone with diabetes has blood sugar levels that are dangerously high or low, they almost always act immediately and the world of care changes.

How do we build that care network? Carefully. First, we must start with the psychology. No one wants to be sick, have a chronic condition, or need "help." As we know from our children, they need help until they become independent, and then they often frustratingly reject any efforts with that phrase every parent knows: "I can do it myself!" Adults feel the same way, only more so. And this gets worse, not better, as people age. Many elderly people will forgo care rather than ask for a ride to the physician's office, for example. What we need to build is an "invisible" care network—one that only appears when you need it and does so in ways that are additive in value. Rather than build a system of health coaches who randomly call, we must empower informed, connected health consumers to build their own care teams and set the parameters of when they want information shared on their need for support and with whom. They are now in charge of their care, and we need to welcome that.

> "What we need to build is an 'invisible' care network."

Chirine provided a solution I needed and we both laughed about it. It was timely, positive, and valuable. As I explained, at that moment, she knew what my body needed better than I did, all while sitting at her desk, which illustrates the potential of a whole new kind of support for people with chronic conditions. A system where your personal care team (starting with the people around you) understands that you may occasionally need some support, knows how to provide it, and offers real-time care. It also highlighted an important factor in the equation of better health: people with chronic conditions don't just need information and care to achieve better outcomes, but they also need to feel supported and encouraged in the right way to deal with a condition that can often seem frustrating and draining. The impact of chronic conditions transcends the physiological factors of health to affect the psychological aspects of living. This emphasizes the importance of treating not only the condition and the underlying behavior that causes it but also the mental and social experiences that accompany it.

Chronic conditions can be inherently isolating. To live with one means to lose something important to you: the freedom of eating without restrictions, of not following a strict set of rules, of existing beyond the shadow of uncertainty and sometimes fear. Meanwhile, those surrounding you—whether intentionally or unintentionally—may remind you of the freedoms you are no longer able to enjoy. Each instance can serve to isolate people with chronic conditions by making them feel different from others who don't need to deal with hypertension, depression, diabetes, heart disease, or obesity. Over time, these reminders accumulate, and without support to alleviate their impact, they negatively influence the path toward better health. All too often, people get frustrated and simply withdraw.

The traditional health-care system often makes people feel more alone. Once people enter the health-care system, they often lose the respect and power afforded to them in every other aspect of their lives. People with chronic conditions can feel less like a person than a condition when they become a patient, in part because health-care providers treat them as a condition. For instance, people with diabetes are often referred to as "diabetics" inside and outside the health-care system, by people who should know better. People with chronic conditions also lose control of their interactions and experiences, and physicians issue reprimands when people don't adhere to treatments. Again, they are often treating the condition using a standardized protocol and not the person, who is an individual with unique needs and circumstances. All this comes as the result of health-care providers lacking information, time, and context to offer personalized support and attention to the whole person and to build a real sense of trust. Our health system is not convenient, is time consuming, and often doesn't make you feel better—either emotionally or physically. It's no surprise that many people who have the most serious challenges with their chronic conditions often avoid the system until their health reaches a critical state, giving them no alternative but to seek out the most expensive care available.

Traditional disease management programs have not done much

"Informed, connected health consumers already leverage the power of the internet."

better in supporting people with chronic conditions than traditional health care. While well intentioned, these programs also fail to provide the support people need when they need it (in context) and only when they need it. And generalized coaches, because we have asked them to do everything, often do not do anything well. Everyone with a chronic condition has a story about the call they received at work or home at the most inappropriate and least desirable time by someone who really can't help them in any case. Failing to recognize the context and timing of the interaction, the call itself adds to the hassle of having a chronic condition in the first place. Without the ability to offer an experience that is context aware or personalized, traditional disease management programs invariably take an outside-in approach to support that overlooks the psychological issues, challenges, and stresses of having a chronic condition. Ultimately, they neglect the factors crucial to one's psychological well-being.

91

To understand the need to build a supportive network for those affected by chronic conditions, look no further than online forums and blogs. Informed, connected health consumers already leverage the power of the internet to tap into communities of like-minded people affected by the same

> **"New solutions already exist that leverage the power of online communities."**

chronic conditions. People use these outlets to exchange information vital to their care but also to feel a sense of community and unity with those dealing with similar challenges. In many ways, these online forums represent a response to the lack of support people receive from participants in the traditional health-care system. They demonstrate the strong desire people feel for a more shared experience. And it doesn't just include people with chronic conditions but family and friends that make up the personal care team of those affected. People want the autonomy to control their own health-care decisions and how that is shared with others, but at the same time, they want to feel a part of a collective body, where everyone is working toward shared goals and outcomes. To see that passion in action, attend any fundraiser for any chronic condition. It's amazing what happens.

New solutions already exist that leverage the power of online communities to create a more social and supportive

92

experience. PatientsLikeMe is a perfect example. The Massachusetts-based company hosts an online community that unites more than 500,000 people with chronic and other life-threatening conditions. Using the platform, people share their health information and experiences to support others dealing with heart disease, diabetes, obesity, and other equally serious conditions, like cancer. PatientsLikeMe provides an outlet for people to become more knowledgeable about their condition as well as feel more connected to others dealing with similar problems. And it also enables people to feel more satisfied in offering support to others who need it. Now, PatientsLikeMe is beginning to use the power of shared information and data science to develop better solutions. It captures and synthesizes a variety of information contributed over the network to provide more personalized, targeted recommendations for those using the platform.

Imagine if after being diagnosed, instead of another coaching program, your physician told you the top three sites for a community of "patients like you" so you would know what to expect. And imagine they provided you with emails to explain your condition to everyone who needed to know, in understandable terms, as well as invitations for people to join your own support network that looked like invitations to a wedding, the commitments needed from them, what they should do, etc. It would create a whole new experience with new empathy and understanding that the real challenge begins once someone is diagnosed—not just physically but emotionally.

PatientsLikeMe serves as a strong and important step in the right direction. A strong community is only part of what someone with a chronic condition needs to be successful in managing and improving their health. PatientsLikeMe provides a valuable piece of the experience but does not address the total experience of living with a chronic condition. We need a solution that does.

Creating Your Own Personal Care Team

The personal care team serves as the most important, reliable, immediate, and least expensive source of support for those dealing with a chronic condition. According to Dr. Polonsky, the personal care team drives better outcomes: "In behavioral psychology, one of the things we know across the board is, most people always do better when they have someone in their life rooting for them, whether that means someone willing to make lifestyle changes with you or show you they care."

> **"Family and friends don't understand how we feel beyond what we tell them."**

Despite the important role family and friends play in our

lives, our personal care teams lack awareness of the *body's vital narrative*—the ability to really know what's going on at any given time, be there at the right time to help, and know what to do. All three have to come together to make the interaction valuable and effective. Family and friends don't understand how we feel beyond what we tell them. Sometimes we don't care to tell them, and other times we can't, at least not precisely. If they truly knew, they could provide the most appropriate assistance immediately. For instance, our friends would offer comfort and support if they knew we experienced a difficult day. While our personal care teams (family, friends, spouses, roommates) understand us best and care about us most, we need to connect them so they can help and empower them so they know what help we need and when we need it.

When it comes to chronic conditions, the personal care team provides considerable value for many reasons. First, when you post your health goals and tell your friends about them, you are 50 percent more likely to achieve them.[22] Why? On the one hand, they can now remind you of your objectives and help you make them a daily priority. On the other, we naturally feel a sense of accountability for achieving our goals because we don't want to disappoint those we care about, especially when it comes to our perceived commitment to our health. While we may easily justify skipping a healthy activity to ourselves, it becomes far more complicated, important,

---

[22] Jackie Coleman, and John Coleman. "Increase the Odds of Achieving Your Goals by Setting Them with Your Spouse." *Harvard Business Review*. February 3, 2015. Accessed June 11, 2018. https://hbr.org/2015/02/increase-the-odds-of-achieving-your-goals-by-setting-them-with-your-spouse

and consequential to us when we must justify the behavior to someone else. The personal care team brings the power to keep us focused on our goals, and motivate us to achieve them, while limiting the perceived difficulty of obstacles that may detract from our progress. Family and friends also influence our behavior through theirs. Growing up, we all heard our parents talk about the importance of not hanging out with the "wrong crowd." Why? Because we tend to adopt similar behaviors to those with whom we socialize. And now there is a bevy of scientific research to support that idea. If we spend time with people who don't exercise, the behavior becomes less important to us. Alternatively, if we socialize with people who value fitness, we likely adopt fitness as a priority. The same holds true for managing chronic conditions. If the people closest to us (both in relationships and also in proximity) understand our health goals, they will support behaviors that make it easier to manage a chronic condition. For example, everything from exercise to the choice of restaurants (that might offer a broader menu with healthier food) can support our personal goals, but only if people know them. This can provide the benefit of making people with chronic conditions feel less isolated, and more supported, while switching their focus from the difficulty of

> **"If we socialize with people who value fitness, we likely adopt fitness as a priority."**

the task to the social interaction. In turn, the personal care team can foster greater motivation and accountability to engage in healthier behaviors. What better way to promote positive health than by surrounding yourself with friends and family who know what your goals are and want you to succeed?

> "The personal care team serves as one of the best indicators of how well people with chronic conditions will do in the right environment."

The more we can empower your personal care team with real-time, context-aware, personalized information, the better support family and friends can provide when people need it most, such as when they feel most insecure and sensitive about their chronic conditions. High blood sugar may prevent someone from engaging in physical activity, which in a social setting, may cause the individual to feel disheartened and even embarrassed. But imagine the power of providing real-time, context-aware, personalized information to his or her friends so they can empathize and recommend a different activity.

I've seen this firsthand with my son Sam playing basketball with his friends. In cases where his blood sugar was too high or too low, he had to stop playing. And I watched his friends say they were tired too and suggest doing something else . . . usually eating. This fundamentally changed some of the negativity of living with a chronic condition, and it has nothing to do with medications or physicians or physiology. It's all social and about the care team—that team of people who immediately surround you in your everyday life. The flip side? Once, a coach who didn't know that Sam had Type 1 Diabetes yelled at him for "dogging it" and not putting out full effort. It wasn't the coach's fault. He simply didn't have the information.

The personal care team serves as one of the best indicators of how well people with chronic conditions will do in the right environment. The more involved, supportive, and caring the personal care team, the better people perform from a physiological and psychological standpoint. While the traditional health-care system does nothing to boost the power of this team to support those affected, we need to leverage this important asset to carry some of the burden of living with a chronic condition.

Leveraging the Support of Certified Diabetes Educators

We also need to expand the network to include clinical support available whenever and wherever people with chronic conditions need it if medical questions arise. Certified diabetes educators (CDEs) represent a perfect example of a comprehensive supportive network for people with diabetes.

Certified diabetes educators are licensed in at least one of several clinical disciplines—clinical psychology, nursing, or pharmacy, or as dietitians, to name a few—and require two years of professional experience. They also need 1,000 hours of hands-on experience educating and caring for people with prediabetes or diabetes before they can attain their CDE certification. The experience and knowledge these professionals acquire will, in many cases, make them more capable than a physician in helping people with chronic conditions achieve better outcomes. While CDEs provide value through delivering the real-time care people with diabetes need, they also provide significant value by offering psychological and emotional support. For people with diabetes, there is a lot of comfort that comes from knowing someone is always prepared to respond when they need it. The feeling of comfort also comes from eliminating the fear and uncertainty of a critical health event, of finding oneself alone when their condition makes them most vulnerable. Comfort comes from knowing they are always connected to a human voice that can provide the information

99

"For people with diabetes, there is a lot of comfort that comes from knowing someone is always prepared to respond when they need it."

and recommendations they need to get better. Who hasn't thought, "I wish I could talk to someone right now who knows

CHAPTER 5: BUILDING A CARING COMMUNITY

the answer to this question"? While CDEs care for people by providing recommendations, information, and awareness, they also offer support in the form of empathy and treating people as people rather than a "condition." Chronic conditions take away something very important to those affected by them—the simple freedoms that they enjoyed at some other point in their lives. For people with diabetes, it means the freedom of eating without worrying about blood glucose or pricking their finger several times a day or simply feeling well enough to participate in daily activities that most people would consider normal. CDEs understand the importance of empowering people to feel capable of improving their health on their terms. They don't call or perceive a person with diabetes as a "diabetic" like many health-care professionals do—reducing them to their condition rather than a person affected by one. They also don't take a traditional approach to care—i.e., "This is what you need to get better." Instead, they address people as consumers just as any good business would do: "How can I help?" They understand that treating people as patients turns into a losing game in the fight against chronic conditions. No one wants to become their condition and be told what to do—when, where, and how. Everyone wants recognition and respect. A phone call from a CDE can enable people to better understand what interventions they need to stay healthy as well as cause those affected to feel more comfortable, protected, and encouraged about their chronic conditions.

Redefining the Role of the Health-Care Provider

Since managing a chronic condition is a 24/7/365 activity, it shouldn't come as a surprise that physicians start with a disadvantage, having only limited time to interact with their "patient." To be successful, we need to redefine the physician's role in the health-care system. First, we need to offer physicians access to a broader set of information about the people with chronic conditions in their panel. This is not just a static metric like an A1C test, which understandably was the best we could do when it became the standard, but rather metrics like time-in-range, which provide valuable data on how the body is actually doing managing the disease as well as how the person is doing managing the disease. Both are critical for success. The psychological support needed for people with chronic conditions requires time, information, and context, which physicians currently lack in today's model of care. Information and context, for instance, remain limited to the few minutes physicians can spend learning about each patient and the data they can see in medical records, and today, most medical records don't even have a place to adequately represent the breadth of data from a typical three-month period, let alone turn that data into useful and actionable information. Fifteen minutes is far too short a period to understand the psychological challenges and pressures people face in dealing with their chronic conditions, especially since most of that time must be spent on treating the physical, rather than the mental and emotional, aspects of health. The results are treatments that do not ease the burden of living with a chronic condition, fail to offer empathy and support, and often simply are not effective.

According to Dr. Polonsky, health-care providers are so profoundly limited with the time they have available that many tend to focus singularly on problems, which often works in acute cases but is suboptimal for chronic conditions. For chronic conditions, this overshadows opportunities to recognize progress, which is a critical need in the ongoing effort to manage a chronic condition. People can easily feel ashamed, overwhelmed, and discouraged, especially when health-care providers spend all their time identifying readings considered high or low. Dr. Polonsky teaches health-care providers to take a different approach during their quarterly visits with patients. Rather than take a judgmental approach to blood glucose readings, he instructs health-care providers to help patients recognize what is safe versus unsafe. This focuses the interaction on education rather than judgment.

"A physician should focus on broad trending, for both the population and the person."

Technology now promises to provide physicians with the time, context, and information to more effectively support patients on their journey toward better health. A physician should focus on broad trending, for both the population and the person. And then they need to spend time on the behavioral side of the equation, but often they simply are not allocated the necessary time. We need to provide physicians with better tools that

"For the new model to work, physicians need to embrace a team effort."

will allow them to address the physical issues when a person with diabetes or hypertension presents, but also we need to teach them to understand the patient's experience and context. They need to understand and manage their patients more as people and less as bundles of symptoms. This new model of care and support ensures physicians embrace a role far more meaningful and rewarding for them and their patients.

For the new model to work, physicians need to embrace a team effort where they provide the suggested medical treatment in the context of the person as an individual and then rely on a support team who can provide the empathy and support that is required to truly manage a whole person challenged with one or more chronic conditions. One example of this is Dr. Rushika Fernandopulle, cofounder of Iora Health, who uses a blended model as a central philosophy when recruiting talent for his organization.[23] Dr. Fernandopulle doesn't focus

---

[23] *From the Ground Up*. Boston: Iora Health, 2016. Accessed November 8, 2017. http://online.pubhtml5. com/lcuv/bkxo/

his efforts on recruiting the hard skills or clinical expertise needed for his organization—that can be taught and learned. Instead, he focuses on recruiting people with qualities they possess naturally, such as empathy, kindness, and compassion to others. These are the qualities that are essential to treating patients as people and consumers. His philosophy remains a consistent value point for Iora Health, which provides primary care services to those dealing with chronic conditions. The company takes a value-based approach to care by focusing on the needs of individual patients while providing a solution that results in more affordable, sustainable, and effective care at the population level. The future calls for more health-care providers to embrace this focus on empathy and support rather than relying solely on clinical "fixes."

Building a Caring Community of Informed, Connected Health Consumers

Earlier in this chapter, we explored the example of PatientsLikeMe to illustrate the power of connection. Websites such as PatientsLikeMe offer value not only in the information they provide but also through the sense of community and intimacy they foster, by reassuring people they are not alone. No supportive network would be complete without combining and leveraging the unique experiences and information of people managing chronic conditions. However, today, we can begin to realize the untapped potential of this network by leveraging the ability to connect both people and data—or better said, information.

To illustrate the structure and dynamic of this network, consider the example of Waze, technology that drivers use to help each other navigate by using real-time information about traffic and road conditions. This solution, in the form of a social platform, learns from individual drivers and populations to produce optimal value. Notice that I said, "that drivers use to help each other." Initially, many people using Waze didn't realize that while we benefit as recipients of information that reduces our travel time, we also become a contributor to the network. We send personal alerts to educate others about our experiences, such as if we see an accident or if road conditions become hazardous. We engage in these actions so others learn from our experience to improve theirs. We also become one node among thousands supplying information back to the network about traffic conditions, providing a variety of metrics from how fast we travel to how many stops we make, all without doing anything at all. We constantly contribute and receive this feedback, which the network captures, collects, and

> "We engage in these actions so others learn from our experience to improve theirs."

synthesizes. The volume of information exchanged on the platform enables Waze to make us smarter without us even knowing about it while, at the same time, providing a social outlet so we feel connected to people like us. The more people who use Waze, the better we can understand traffic patterns, opening the door to preventative solutions—like alternative routes—that save people time and headaches on the road.

> "People with diabetes would receive real-time recommendations about future behaviors."

We need to build a similar supportive network for those managing chronic conditions, a network that enables users to share their experiences, while learning from individuals and populations to provide more personalized, context-aware, and preventative solutions. In this new model, people with chronic conditions become active contributors and recipients of information that addresses not just the physiological factors they need to stay healthy but the psychological factors too. This would enable people to feel connection to a community of people like them—in getting help and supplying support—while also serving as contributors and recipients of information about their *body's vital narrative* to inform better solutions for everyone connected. This can all be done without violating personal privacy. In fact, the individual should always be in charge of his or her data. Consider the value of this network, not only in the information it provides but also in the satisfaction, encouragement, motivation, and confidence it would create for those affected by chronic conditions. People with diabetes would receive real-time recommendations about future behaviors that produce the best outcomes for people of their age group, ethnicity, gender, and other characteristics. By personalizing the recommendation, the system invariably increases the likelihood that people feel more motivated, encouraged, and willing to follow the recommendations it provides. That said, once people discover the behavior improves how they feel, provides a sense of accomplishment from completing a task, and demonstrates they can make a difference in their health, the more self-reinforcing it becomes.

The Future of a Caring Community

Building a supportive network of people serves as a necessary and critical driver of better health for informed, connected health consumers. This means developing a system that addresses not just the physiological but also the psychological factors that cause people to experience insecurities and anxieties over their chronic condition. Chronic conditions pose social problems for those who live with them, which calls for social solutions. While support exists today in the form of outreach from personal care teams and online forums, the opportunity now exists to not only expand this support but also empower the people at the other end of the line or the keyboard with the objective science of the *body's vital narrative*, which allows for better, more personalized insights. Using sophisticated innovations, we now stand fully capable of addressing the factors that create the need for support in the first place while also improving the effectiveness of how we encourage and empathize with people who deal with these chronic conditions every day. Building a stronger, more informed, and more expansive network of people serves as another critical component of improving how we manage health at the population level. By empowering individuals to build their own supportive network on their terms—not ours—we ensure they remain active contributors and recipients of information that expands our knowledge about chronic conditions to develop far better solutions than we see today.

• • •

Chapter Summary

- "Chronic conditions pose social problems for those who live with them, which calls for social solutions."

- "While support exists today in the form of outreach from personal care teams and online forums, the opportunity now exists to not only expand this support but also empower the people at the other end of the line or the keyboard with the objective science of the *body's vital narrative*, which allows for better, more personalized insights."

- "Rather than build a system of health coaches who randomly call, we must empower informed, connected health consumers to build their own care teams and set the parameters of when they want information shared on their need for support and with whom. They are now in charge of their care, and we need to welcome that."

CHAPTER 6:
DELIVERING REAL-TIME, CONTEXT-AWARE CARE

You never change things by fighting the existing reality. To change something, build a new model that makes the existing model obsolete."

:: Richard Buckminster Fuller

D iabetes, the fastest-growing chronic condition in the world, touches more than 32 million[24] people across the United States. And diabetes comes in two very different types. Type 1 Diabetes (or T1D) is genetic. People with Type 1 Diabetes don't produce insulin—the hormone that regulates glucose. Without insulin, their cells can't convert glucose into energy, and without energy, their organs can't function. People with Type 1 Diabetes need insulin to survive, so they depend on insulin therapy—self-administering insulin through injections.

For people with Type 1, insulin therapy represents the ongoing process of managing the balance between insulin and glucose in the body at any given time. When blood glucose gets too high, they need to inject themselves with insulin to restore balance. When it falls too low, they need to eat more sugars and carbohydrates to introduce more glucose into their

---

[24] "Statistics About Diabetes." *American Diabetes Association,* last modified July 19, 2017, http://www.diabetes.org/diabetes-basics/statistics/

system. Elevated blood glucose poses long-term risk to the organs, while low levels of glucose pose the short-term risk of a seizure. The problem is, people often can't manage this important balance themselves when levels become too high or too low.

People with diabetes live every day thinking about how to manage this challenge. There is no better example than my son Sam, whom you met earlier in the book. One night at college, he woke up at 4:30 a.m., felt low, checked his blood sugar, and discovered it had fallen critically low, to 37. Blood glucose (or sugar) readings of 90 to 120 are common if you don't have diabetes. Typically, people with diabetes always try to have something like juice close by to immediately raise their blood sugar if it's that low. Sam didn't have anything on his bedside table to raise his blood sugar, and he knew that simply getting out of bed and walking to the refrigerator might trigger a seizure, where the body, to protect itself from running out of energy to power the heart and brain, shuts down all other systems, including walking, talking, etc. Sam wasn't quite sure what he was going to do, and then his phone lit up and began ringing. He answered it only to hear the voice of Kendell on the other end of the line—a certified diabetes educator (CDE) at Livongo who specializes in helping people with diabetes just like Sam during moments of uncertainty or crisis.

"Sam, I see that your blood sugar is 37, which is very low. How can I help?" she asked.

Sam explained the situation—his worry, his past experiences with low readings, and his roommate who would normally help (think care team) but was out for the evening. He was both physically and emotionally alone at that moment.

"I'm right here with you on the phone if you need me, and I'm not going anywhere until we figure this out together," Kendell continued.

They talked through the problem and solution, which included Kendell staying on the phone while Sam rolled out of his bed to get some juice.

The next day, Sam shared the experience with me. He talked through the feeling of being alone that he experienced and the relief from hearing Kendell's calm and reassuring voice on the phone. He also mentioned the sense of safety and protection he felt, knowing that someone would always be there when he needed it. Without Kendell to call him, his only resort would be to call 911 if he couldn't reach someone in the middle of the night—an expensive and embarrassing thing to have to do. Did Sam think of calling his physician or endocrinologist? No, because as we all know, they operate from nine to five. It only reaffirmed my belief in the importance of real-time care, which saves people a considerable amount of cost and pain. Everything turned out OK that night thanks to Kendell, some cool technology, and an understanding of how to really "be there" for someone with a chronic condition. It made me proud to be the CEO of Livongo but also made me wonder why we can't provide this same level of care, of reassurance, of safety, to every person with diabetes.

People hold the greatest power to treat their chronic conditions. However, in most cases today, they also have the least control when their

"To keep people healthy, we must ensure they get real-time care when they need it most."

condition turns critical and renders them the most vulnerable. Empowering the informed, connected health consumer with information and building a caring community serves as part of the change needed to address the chronic-condition epidemic but not the whole solution. To keep people healthy, we must ensure they get real-time care when they need it most. We must embrace a fundamentally different model than what we deem as "care" today—surgery, hospitals, physicians— to provide people with the tools and knowledge they need to regain control over their health conditions. This model of personalized, context-aware care—based entirely on the needs of the individual—is the only viable and sustainable solution to manage the health of individuals like Sam and the populations they represent. It calls for redefining our mental models and expectations of what health and health care can and should look like. And it requires technology to allow us to redesign how people receive and experience care. Smart, connected devices, backed by cloud technology and data

113

science, make it possible to introduce and scale higher-quality care and a more efficient system for those managing chronic conditions when and where they need it, saving them from medical issues, concerns, and costs.

Chronic conditions don't operate according to normal working hours. They don't wait until people see their physician to pose significant health consequences. They also don't alert people before their blood sugar becomes critically high or low, or their blood pressure raises off the charts, or they have an episode of depression, each of which can present significant risks to their health. Instead, chronic conditions strike in the middle of the night, on weekends, or when family and friends leave the house. They strike without warning for those without access to sophisticated tools and a support network always prepared to respond. Events like these become the costliest and most challenging for people with chronic conditions. They pose life-threatening situations as well as psychological and physiological setbacks that can overtake positive momentum toward better health that took months or years to create. They represent the most demoralizing and discouraging events that often can cause people to revert to poor habits and previous

"Unfortunately, the traditional health-care system is not designed to be predictive or preventive but rather treatment oriented."

lifestyles. And they remain almost entirely preventable with responsive, real-time action.

Unfortunately, the traditional health-care system is not designed to be predictive or preventive but rather treatment oriented. It is the most available outlet to people with chronic conditions, but it serves as the most expensive and unsustainable option. The emergency room (the ER) is traditional health care's best answer for managing chronic conditions, illustrating just one of the fundamental flaws of the current model of care. The ER stays open when people with chronic conditions need care, offering service 24/7. Everyone agrees that ERs are not the best solution, clinically or financially. ERs charge people with chronic conditions thousands of dollars to receive the same solutions readily available in the home or at the pharmacy or even, today, by telehealth or through a 24-hour clinic. The solution to restoring blood sugar stays fundamentally the same no matter where people go: the sooner blood sugar is restored to normal levels the better. The existing system simply isn't designed to treat chronic conditions, whether diabetes or any other chronic condition, and because of that, it remains ineffective and expensive.

Health care is a paradox. The more successful we are at keeping people healthy, the longer they live and, therefore, the more health issues they will continue to have. We can't truly "fix" health care, because tomorrow will always call for more of it than we provide today. At the same time, we can't sustain the traditional model of health care today from a cost and care perspective. The status quo won't allow us to meet the challenges of the present, not to mention the future. We must become smarter about the ways we think about and deliver care.

New models in health-care delivery continue to emerge in response to the lack of care available to those who need it. Telehealth serves as a good example of a service that enables patients to meet with their physicians and receive real-time care. In many ways, telehealth is a significant step in the right direction—it makes resources more available when people need them. Today, calling and reaching a family physician is at best difficult and time consuming, and many would say it is impossible. But now using telehealth services such as Teladoc, American Well, or Doctor On Demand, people can "see" a physician within minutes. With nothing more than an internet connection, they can receive medical attention whenever they need it and wherever they are, for a variety of services. Telehealth solves the problem of access to real-time treatment; however, it preserves the idea that you need to talk with a physician to get the best answers

> **"Calling and reaching a family physician is at best difficult and time consuming, and many would say it is impossible."**

to your health-care questions. A better model begins with the assumption that you, equipped with the right information, are in charge of your own care. This is, in fact, the next stage beyond telehealth. New technology provides the context-aware, personalized, preventive care that all people—especially those with chronic conditions—want and need. Telehealth, for instance, doesn't provide physicians or consumers with information or context that makes them smarter about what people need to become healthier. It also doesn't provide all the options—predicting what you will need and prescribing a solution (meds, more exercise, a change in diet, or on occasion, a visit to see a physician)—because the only time people use it occurs after a health event. And it doesn't solve the fundamental problem of whether people need to rely on physicians in the first place. Beyond making the health-care system more consumer focused and convenient, which is both important and necessary, telehealth

"Emerging innovations now promise to provide those affected by chronic conditions with everything they need to stay healthy and protected."

leaves significant room to improve how we empower informed, connected health consumers to stay healthy in the first place and, where necessary, treat and address chronic conditions.

Care is taking on a new definition. Emerging innovations now promise to provide those affected by chronic conditions

CHAPTER 6: DELIVERING REAL-TIME, CONTEXT-AWARE CARE

with everything they need to stay healthy and protected. No longer does it just mean surgery, or hospitals, or physicians but also information, access, choice, support, and an awareness of the cost of each option, which in itself is a quality issue. No sense prescribing expensive drugs to patients who can't afford them, and that is no longer just under-resourced populations because, given the cost

> "The new model of care recognizes that the best solution depends on the individual and his or her context."

of new treatments, it can be almost anyone. The new definition of care calls for creating context-aware solutions that optimize a person's health at the current moment. And only that individual, that person, really knows what the perfect solution is for them in the moment. Perhaps a good analogy is what I call the banana problem. If you are sent to the store to pick up some bananas and you see only overripe ones, should you buy them? The question can only be answered if you know the context. If they are to be used for banana bread, that's great. If they are for a fruit salad, you need to try another store. But no one at the store can make the choice for you and hope to be right. Health care runs into this problem in spades because health care is as personal as it gets.

Care may be a text message delivered immediately to someone's smartphone or a voice from someone knowledgeable about chronic conditions and what's happening with your body at that moment in time. As a next level, care can be delivered by the kind of community we explored in chapter five. And it can also take shape as the helping hand of a family member or friend, or a connection through a community of people who share the same challenge and whom you may have never met before. The new model of care recognizes that the best solution depends on the individual and his or her context. It doesn't call for a standard answer for everyone or even a planned solution, such as a quarterly visit to the doctor's office, which contrary to old beliefs, is an enormously inefficient use of our talented physicians. It calls for recognizing that the kind of care people need now can change moments later. The new model approaches health as the incredibly nuanced system it is. It is all about personalization for effectiveness with an N of 1.

To illustrate the need for context-aware care, consider another example commonly used by the Young Presidents' Organization (YPO) in their leadership training for chief executives and business leaders around the world. YPO starts by setting the scene: You are riding the bus home from work when a woman and her children board at one of the stops. The children begin running back and forth down the aisle, yelling, and acting unruly. After minutes pass, you decide to speak up. You gesture to the woman to get her attention and say, "Would you please take care of your kids?"

"I'm so sorry," she responds. "We're returning from the hospital. They just lost their father."

> **"They should feel confident that there is always access to care and support, but only when they believe it's necessary."**

Now, consider how this new information would change your perspective. Would you still see the behavior of the children as inappropriate? Would you still judge the mother? Of course not. You would see any behavior as appropriate, given the circumstances. YPO teaches this example to illustrate an important lesson: actions and events don't occur in a vacuum. Rather, they occur in a certain context, which adds meaning to them. Without recognizing the context, we could make assumptions and judgments that prove to be inaccurate, sometimes false, and even damaging. To provide the best care, we must develop a full understanding of people's health now to provide only the best and most appropriate solutions possible. That includes social determinants of health, such as income, family situation, and stress factors. To truly deliver effective care, we have to understand and treat the whole person.

Today, the innovations empowering the informed, connected health consumer with information also promise to unlock a new model of context-aware care for those affected—a model like OnStar introduced in chapter three. Drivers who get into an accident don't need to wait for an appointment to get the care they need. Once the sensor is triggered, OnStar provides assistance immediately. OnStar delivers support that transcends the boundaries of time, space, and context to improve outcomes and save lives. We need to create a similar model for chronic conditions. When people find themselves most vulnerable to manage their chronic conditions, they should get the care they need to take back control of their health. They should feel confident that there is always access to care and support, but only when they believe it's necessary. Just as OnStar provides a human voice to aid drivers after a crash, specialists in chronic conditions provide remote care to those affected at times they need support. And just as OnStar deploys assistance at the appropriate location, the personal care team intervenes at the appropriate time and location.

Leveraging 24/7 Responsive Service from Certified Diabetes Educators

Recall the story of Sam at the start of the chapter. Several elements made the real-time care he received possible. First, he needed a connected device to reliably transmit his blood glucose readings in real time—not a Bluetooth device that he would have to synch but an always-on cellular connection.

Second, Kendell, his CDE, needed a platform to view those results as well as data analytics to diagnose his health status and alert her and Sam's care network. Third, she needed a way to get in contact with him, so she used the one device that virtually all of us carry everywhere to communicate: a smartphone. All these variables are necessary to enable this kind of support—a call to my son within 90 seconds, before his health could become an issue requiring an expensive intervention—and they are increasingly being offered across many chronic conditions. This is the future of health and health care. But there is one more requirement.

Perhaps most important, the model required Kendell, a new kind of health professional capable of providing the care that results in the best outcomes for those affected by chronic conditions. As a CDE, Kendell specializes in helping people like Sam stay healthy. In chapter five, we explored the certification requirements of CDEs. In Kendell's case, she became licensed as a certified dietitian, specializing in the clinical nutrition critical to Sam's health. In contrast, the average medical student only receives several days of training over a multiyear degree. She also accumulated over 1,000 hours of experience providing care to people with diabetes. So the most qualified person to treat Sam may not be the one with the most degrees or education but rather a combination of the most empathetic, best problem solver with expertise in the specific condition someone is dealing with at that time. Would

Kendell be the right person for someone dealing with Crohn's disease? Probably not, but in the future, people dealing with Crohn's should expect to talk with an expert on the phone if that's their issue. And we can be that good.

The good news is that Kendell knew how to most effectively deal with Sam's blood sugar, given his unique history—recorded on her screen—and his patterns of high and low blood sugar levels, as well as how to interact with him to ensure he remained calm and capable of improving his situation. She understood how to diagnose the signs when people can and cannot care for themselves. This enhanced training, information, and emotional intelligence is necessary because the interaction took place remotely, not within the controlled environment of a health-care facility or even a face-to-face interaction where nonverbal cues provide additional information to those delivering care. It required a knowledge base and skill set far different from what our medical schools produce today. And because only this type of model works to ensure entire populations of people managing chronic conditions receive the care they need when and where they need it, the demand for certified diabetes educators like Kendell will only continue to grow as we seek to personalize care at scale.

We will need to rethink and redesign how we train an entire workforce tasked with caring for informed, connected health consumers. There is no longer an information advantage or imbalance but rather a skill set derived from specific education and experience and software to connect the right people to the right skills at exactly the right time.

We can no longer expect physicians to be experts on every medical condition, but we should expect expert care for every issue we have. Rather than rely on physicians to treat all our problems, we should look to them for guidance and information on how to get the best care we need. Increasingly, physicians are shifting away from their traditional role as all-knowing, all-purpose health-care professionals to counselors who help us sort through the complexity of medical care and options today. This new role calls for physicians to no longer attempt to be the experts on every problem they encounter. Rather, they research issues side by side with us, bringing to bear their expertise to help us navigate our options. This represents an important evolution, ensuring informed, connected health consumers receive better care that reflects the expectations they hold in every other aspect of their lives. If we visited a computer repair technician to fix our PC, for instance, we would expect the technician to direct us to another vendor if he or she only specialized in fixing Apple computers. Yet in health care, some physicians attempt to solve every problem

"Some physicians attempt to solve every problem rather than refer us to the best resources."

rather than refer us to the best resources, which can prevent us from getting the best care possible. In the past, physicians would research problems to inform a better solution. Today, they lack the time to investigate each and every patient issue— and they don't get reimbursed to perform that work. As a result, physicians often don't know the best answer and can only provide us with the best solution they can develop in the 15 minutes allotted to a visit. This often means we fail to get the care we need.

Just as care is taking on a new definition, so is the person providing it. Today's challenges require a new role in the health-care environment: a professional who serves as an educator in the fight against chronic conditions, a navigator through the system, and a counselor. Unlike traditional physicians, educators provide care in the form of information and awareness, not invasive procedures. They will focus on empowering consumers with information, transparency, and control. OnStar doesn't demand anything from drivers after a crash or try to dictate their experience—nor should we when people with chronic conditions need care.

That night in Sam's apartment, Kendell demonstrated the approach we need to take with informed, connected health consumers. On her computer, she could diagnose his *body's vital narrative* in real time, seeing the health patterns that led to the current moment. She could also see the physiological factors that made Sam and his chronic condition unique. Still, she didn't know beyond what she could see on her computer screen, such as his exact location, whether he was alone, or what food and juice he had in his apartment. She needed to rely on him just as Sam relied on her. It became a real-time collaboration, borne out of mutual respect for what the other could bring to the table. Kendell knew, just as Sam did, that the best outcome depended on working together, a relationship every successful enterprise fosters with its customers.

Empowering the Personal Care Team to Deliver Real-Time Care

Despite the real-time care she gave Sam, Kendell couldn't provide him with physical care. She could speak to him and talk him through his adverse health event, she could even call an ambulance if needed, but she still couldn't open the refrigerator and bring him juice. The new system requires people like Kendell to succeed, but it also requires more to complete the ecosystem of real-time care: a personal care team. Comprised of family, friends, and those around people with chronic conditions, the personal care team provides the least expensive, most reliable, and most immediate care of anyone, and most importantly, it offers the ability to physically care for loved ones when needed. For people with chronic conditions, the personal care team evolves with them as their lives and responsibilities change over time. No matter what this change looks like, the personal care team always includes people who care for those affected. Chronic conditions live with people 24/7, and that means that the primary and most effective and efficient caregivers are the people physically closest to the person with a chronic condition. Additionally, these people often have the most context. How often have you heard a friend or family member say, "That would never work for (fill in the blank)"?

For Sam, his care team started as his mother and me. When he grew older, it became his brother and sister. Soon after, it evolved into his friends, teachers, college roommates, coaches, and teammates. As the care team changed and expanded, we needed to educate newcomers about what Sam needed to stay healthy—including the warning signs of when he needed care, how they should respond, etc. We talked to his friends, instructed his teachers. Ensuring that the people around Sam remained prepared to respond to his needs kept him, and continues to keep him, healthy. The only change is that Sam now is in charge of his care team, educating them and ensuring they are there for him if needed. And Sam has one advantage previously unavailable: 24-hour coverage

> "The personal care team cannot always prevent the worst from happening."

from Livongo.

Despite its importance, today, the personal care team almost always lacks the tools to remain context aware and prepared to assist those closest to them with chronic conditions. Family and friends rely on instinct and observation to diagnose when loved ones need care. Yet this only proves effective when they are present and focused on the person with the chronic condition. It doesn't solve the problem of what happens when they are not around or not paying attention. Even when family members sit in another room, they can't predict and respond to their loved one's needs without knowledge of his or her *body's vital narrative* at that point in time. The personal care team cannot always prevent the worst from happening. But with better tools, they can respond immediately when those affected need their care. Take the example of Ginger.io, a company providing an innovative solution for those fighting depression, anxiety, and stress. The Silicon Valley-based enterprise provides a smartphone app that tracks cell phone habits to detect behavior change, which serves as a key indicator of depression. People who become depressed may stop making phone calls, after usually making a certain number a day, for instance. Or they may stay in bed,

> "The human and financial costs of this scenario could be devastating for everyone involved."

in which case their phone never moves. As we explored earlier, people rely on their smartphones as a necessary tool in their lives. We carry one wherever we go and use it for everything from banking to social media to entertainment. Ginger.io is another innovative company transforming the tools people readily use in their daily lives into personalized, scalable solutions that can address chronic conditions more cost effectively and sustainably.

In chapter four, we explored the example of someone experiencing a diabetic seizure while driving a car. The human and financial costs of this scenario could be devastating for everyone involved, but they are highly preventable with knowledge of the warning signs hidden in the *body's vital narrative*. With near-real-time and real-time remote monitoring, we believe we can prevent nearly eight out of every ten cases in which people experience a seizure. For instance, a simple alert delivered to the personal care team can ensure that family members and friends help with the management of chronic conditions immediately

"This intervention works because drivers value their family and friends, and feel accountable to them."

when needed. They can, for instance, stop a loved one from driving to the grocery store to get food when his or her blood glucose falls too low, and instead make the trip themselves.

An analogous example occurs when family and friends prevent loved ones from drinking and driving. They intervene by taking the keys from the intoxicated person before he or she can get on the road. This intervention works because drivers value their family and friends, and feel accountable to them; after all, the personal care team remains a close and important group protecting drivers' best interests. The entire "Friends Don't Let Friends Drive Drunk" campaign requires a close community of people who surround us because they know us best. The solution does not require contacting our physicians, who lack any information and context about what we need at the time to stay healthy and safe. Whatever the context, the personal care team can provide the kind of care the situation demands, shouldering the burden of managing the condition long enough for those affected to regain control over their health. In many ways, context-aware information enables the personal care team to rewind the clocks on the most expensive and debilitating events that people with chronic conditions experience. Something as simple as a text message can mean the difference between a life-threatening injury and minor hiccup in the journey toward better health. As an example, we were made aware, through Facebook, of someone on the Livongo network who received

> **"The new model of chronic care combines the efforts of CDEs with those of the personal care team."**

a text message after his elderly mother's blood sugar reached critically high levels. He received the message in time, tried to contact her, and then drove to her home, only to find her collapsed on the floor. Had he not become aware through the text message sent to alert him to her condition—very high blood sugar—the consequences would have almost certainly been the loss of her life. Fortunately, he ensured his mother received the care she needed. Every person with chronic conditions deserves this kind of safety net to keep them safe and protected.

The new model of chronic care combines the efforts of CDEs with those of the personal care team. It alerts not only people like Kendell to provide assistance but also immediate family and friends. It combines the knowledge and expertise of the medical establishment (i.e., endocrinologists, physicians, and certified diabetes educators) with the immediate, physical intervention of those also experienced in living with chronic illness on a day-to-day basis. Using this model, we create a hierarchy of skill, care, and cost. For the same reasons Kendell contacts people with chronic conditions on their smartphones, the personal care team receives real-time alerts by text message, email, or whatever way is easiest.

Empowering the personal care team with information— the same information that empowers the informed, connected health consumer—leads to better care. Issues related to someone's chronic condition can still send people into

131

distress, but the outcome doesn't need to become as devastating, disruptive, or expensive as is often the case today.

Keeping Health-Care Providers Informed

On quarterly visits to their health-care providers, people with diabetes often watch as their physicians painfully rifle through the full log of their blood glucose readings over the past three months. Physicians must decipher and synthesize hundreds of numbers within minutes to inform their medical advice and recommendations, assuming the patient even has them. There are two things wrong with this interaction. First, physicians can't realistically provide an accurate assessment, given the lack of information, too much information, or amount of time allotted during a routine visit. The numbers represent nothing more than data, providing no correlation to the lifestyle behaviors or factors that ultimately produced them, forcing physicians to rely on patients to provide context that invariably leads to imprecise and incomplete information. Second, there is no reason that people should be asked to see their physician quarterly, unless they need to, and this should and can now be determined remotely, by someone reviewing the health consumer's results before the appointment is ever scheduled. The current traditional model of care wastes physicians' time by asking them to do more than they reasonably can and wastes patients' time by requiring them to visit a physician's office when their health might be perfectly fine, taking important spots that could be used to treat people who really do need care.

A far better model would be to begin by only scheduling those who really need care, based on remote monitoring and analysis of not just the numbers but the numbers in the context of a person's *vital narrative*: their environment, their exercise and eating patterns, changes, and many other factors we can now consider in a true health assessment. And then we have to deliver and prepare our most valuable assets, our physicians, not just with data and numbers but with valuable information to inform a visit and help them manage both a population (their panel) and a person.

This is the model we are fast at work building today! And the Centers for Medicare and Medicaid Services (CMS), by recently putting into place reimbursement codes for remotely monitoring people with two or more chronic conditions, is paving the way. However, for this to work, physicians need access to information— not just data—about

"However, for this to work, physicians need access to information."

the ongoing health state of those with chronic conditions, including when health patterns turn critical and require medical care. This would enable physicians to provide the best judgment, direction, and guidance to determine the most appropriate care plan for the population and each individual member of it. It would also enable physicians to understand how and when to deliver care and to whom. It is a far different model than the traditional one, albeit a more meaningful and valuable one with regard to allocating the right (and often scarce and expensive) resources where they matter most.

Some years ago, before the United States normalized relations with Cuba, I traveled there to learn about Cuba's health-care system. It turns out that while generally considered poor and without resources, Cuba has an effective model for managing the health of their population. In the community clinics I visited, for every physician, they employed roughly 10 nurses and 25 care coordinators. This comes from the recognition that well-trained care coordinators can perform most of the care needed by people with chronic conditions, care that physicians sometimes perform in our country or that may not be provided at all. Cuba embraces this model out of necessity— physicians remain too scarce and expensive to meet demand. Yet it also embraces this model because it works: Cuba reports far better outcomes for its people with chronic conditions—all

"We should understand that models, like the one used in Cuba, may face resistance."

its people, not just wealthy ones—than we do in the United States. But how? How does a country with a GDP of roughly $87 billion, compared with our nearly $19 trillion, and with far less technological capability, achieve better results?[25] Answered simply, Cuba has a better-designed model of care—one that combines education and simple interventions to ensure people can better manage their own health.

I'm not suggesting that if you need complex surgery you should go to Cuba, but for chronic conditions, they, in fact, do a better job.[26] Imagine the kind of value we could create by embracing a similar model to what Cuba is practicing, while empowering it with smart innovation available in the United States. Imagine the outcomes we could improve for everyone in the health-care equation and create meaningful employment as well.

To truly address the chronic-care crisis in this country, we must look for innovations everywhere and must be ready to adopt and evaluate them. That said, we should understand that models, like the one used in Cuba, may face resistance from health systems and physicians, fearing they would reduce demand for their services and mean less revenue or simply doubting their effectiveness. This perception, however, is based on the fee-for-service system, which needs to be replaced with a value-based reimbursement plan that rewards

---

[25] "Cuba," The World Bank Group, accessed September 26, 2017, https://data.worldbank.org/country/cuba?view=chart.

[26] C. William Keck, and Gail A. Reed. "The Curious Case of Cuba." *American Journal of Public Health* 102, no. 8 (August 2012), Accessed June 6, 2018. DOI: 10.2105/AJPH.2012.300822

both health systems and physicians for keeping people healthy. And if that model is truly embraced, and if a value-based system was adopted, ensuring physicians spent their time treating patients who needed their care versus those who don't, they would actually be able to bill at higher rates, given the complexity of the patients they were seeing, or in even more innovative designs, not bill at all but be compensated for the health of the panel of patients they manage. As the shift toward performance-based reimbursement continues, however slowly, health systems and physicians will all need to make the commitment, both for economic reasons and because it simply delivers better care and better overall population health. And this model will increasingly become the new reality, no matter how anyone feels, whether driven by the government or by business. We can't afford the status quo.

136

Building a Model of Prevention, Not Just Response

The future of health calls for more preventative solutions to chronic conditions, using all of the technology we have, paired with real-time care. Rather than a system focused on addressing problems after the fact, which is too expensive for us to afford, and not good for people, we need to develop a new methodology designed to prevent them from occurring in the first place or, at least, delay and better manage the onset.

This model of predict, prescribe, and prevent is the future of health and care. It is a necessity to manage the health of populations affordably and sustainably, and necessitates the same kind of remote sensing and data science that enables Uptake to help construction companies across the globe predict where equipment will break, using data science, and prescribe preventive maintenance. As we described in chapter three, by sending teams out to do maintenance before the equipment breaks, Uptake reduces or eliminates downtime

"The average is always wrong for everyone."

so companies can stay on schedule, avoid costly bottlenecks, and improve their competitive advantage. The key to Uptake's success begins by learning from equipment on an individual and aggregate (population) level. The system is smart and learns from the sensors installed on the equipment, all of which contribute to the "health state" of a single crane, including how operators use it, how it functions, weather, geography, etc. Uptake uses this information to form a complete understanding of a crane. Then it adds to a growing knowledge base of other cranes around the world and uses data to analyze the unique health states, circumstances, and factors that lead to certain outcomes. By expanding its knowledge on a micro and macro level, it gains a better understanding of the numerous factors that contribute and lead to equipment breakdown. In turn,

137

it develops a personalized recommendation for preventive maintenance for each piece of equipment. Consider this analogy: I used to visit my grandmother, who hardly ever drove her car. Every six months, she would ask me to take her car in for an oil change. Why? The auto industry standard was that everyone should change their oil every six months. How did they determine that? They took an average across the entire population and determined that the typical distance people drove required an oil change every six months. Then they provided a general recommendation. The approach invariably overlooked the most important factors that determined the need for an oil change: how many miles people travel and how hard (at what speeds), and in what kind of traffic the vehicle is driven. While my grandmother rarely drove, I spent considerable time on the road every day. Yet we received the same recommendation, which illustrates the problem with generalized solutions. The average is always wrong for everyone. That's true for your car, but more importantly, it's truer for health care. It makes no more sense to give people a checkup every six months than it does to change the oil in your car. Still, the health-care system continues to operate according to a predetermined schedule that often overlooks the needs of and differences

> **"We need to personalize the solution for care to become much higher quality and more cost effective."**

among people. We need to personalize the solution for care to become much higher quality and more cost effective. We need to begin treating people as well as our equipment!

Using data science, cloud technology, and smart, connected, self-diagnostic devices, we can apply a new kind of informed health model toward managing chronic conditions. One example is empowering CDEs and other health-care professionals to gain new insight into the health patterns that put people at risk, warning those affected of imminent danger, and guiding them through the best solutions to avoid a health crisis. Another may entail sending someone's personal care team real-time alerts that prompt them to act proactively, ensuring that information comes with swift, appropriate, and effective action. A third example may call for sending health-care providers alerts that enable them to focus their efforts on those needing care, understanding their *vital narrative* better and prescribing more proactive treatments for those who would benefit from them. Together, we can build a new model of care that empowers those affected to continue their pursuit of better health, eliminating the factors that impede or detract from their progress. Only then can we begin to transform how we treat chronic

"People with chronic conditions find themselves in need of a new model capable of providing real-time care on their terms to stay healthy."

conditions from after-the-fact attempts to correct a problem or set of problems to the highly manageable process it needs to become in the near future. You've heard the phrase "an accident waiting to happen," and now we can finally prevent it.

While consumers can make intelligent decisions about their health, their condition may affect their ability to manage it alone at certain times. People with chronic conditions find themselves in need of a new model capable of providing real-time care on their terms to stay healthy. We are developing a new model of care that brings together innovations from every other sector of our economy and participants to create a new experience that is absent from the current health-care system today. Rather than base care on observation or a predetermined timetable, we must base it on the hard science of the *body's vital narrative,* empowering individuals with information and the ability to act on the best solutions personalized to their needs at the most appropriate time. We need to also treat those affected by chronic conditions as people and consumers with the intelligence and power to know what they need and put them in charge. The new model of real-time care necessitates that we build a system with better predictive, prescriptive, and preventative capabilities to ensure people with chronic conditions can find and stay on the path to better health.

● ● ●

Chapter Summary

- "People hold the greatest power to treat their chronic conditions. However, in most cases today, they also have the least control when their condition turns critical and renders them the most vulnerable."

- "The new model of chronic care . . . combines the knowledge and expertise of the medical establishment (i.e., endocrinologists, physicians, and certified diabetes educators) with the immediate, physical intervention of those also experienced in living with chronic illness on a day-to-day basis. Using this model, we create a hierarchy of skill, care, and cost."

141

- "Rather than base care on observation or a predetermined timetable, we must base it on the hard science of the *body's vital narrative,* empowering individuals with information and the ability to act on the best solutions personalized to their needs at the most appropriate time."

Chapter 7:
The Innovation Imperative

❝ *You can't outwit fate by standing on the sidelines placing side bets about the outcome of life.*❞

:: Judith McNaught

Recently, I spoke to a large pharmaceutical company about strategic planning. Not long into my talk, someone asked if I could clarify by giving a scenario. So I said, *Here's a scenario. Imagine that your competitor, in your largest and most profitable drug category, announces it will give away all its medications for free on one condition: If it improves behavior, it receives half of the savings earned.* The audience laughed, briefly, until I assured them I was serious. That's the kind of change we can expect in a pay-for-performance, value-based world. Tomorrow won't depend on whether a company produces a great medication but rather if people take it and it makes them healthier. Our challenge is that organizations continue to plan for a future that assumes the current model will continue to exist forever. Except it won't and it can't. While many companies don't see the change coming, others who recognize it are driving toward the cliff that will appear suddenly.

Chicago's taxicabs provide an analogous example.

Tracing their origin as far back as the 1850s, when liveries transported railroad passengers, taxi companies remained confident in their place as the ruler of Chicago's roadways.[27] When ride-sharing services began emerging, they ignored the threat. Rather than compete with the value propositions offered by ride-sharing services—increasing convenience, automating payment, improving the entire experience, etc.— taxicabs adhered to their established model. They continued to charge customers by the mile, while companies like Lyft began charging people for the shortest route to reach their destination, no matter what course drivers took. They believed they were protected and thought ride-sharing services would never be allowed. Eventually, the demand from consumers was too strong, and Chicago's mayor signed an agreement with ride-sharing companies to move their regional offices to the city. Overnight, everything changed. The once-rulers of the roadway continue to see their market share sliding, with taxi revenues declining 40 percent in the last three years alone.[28] And it would have been more, but the new ride-sharing options and the technology they have employed actually made it so convenient that many more people began to use ride-sharing rather than drive, so the market expanded. Change comes quickly. To fight it means to eventually lose, and while embracing it and innovating alongside it doesn't ensure

---

[27] Joshua Lupkin, "Taxis, Liveries, and Limousines," *Encyclopedia of Chicago*, accessed September 28, 2017, http://www.encyclopedia.chicagohistory.org/pages/1232.html

[28] Rachel Koning Beals, "Chicago cab report shows fast-approaching demise at hands of Uber and Lyft." *MarketWatch*, June 06, 2017, http://www.marketwatch.com/story/chicago-cab-report-shows-fast-approaching-demise-at-hands-of-uber-and-lyft-2017-06-06

survival, it gives you the opportunity to play.

The traditional health-care system finds itself in a similar place to the taxi companies in Chicago. Rather than embrace the innovations readily available or emerging in other industries, and make tough choices, the health-care system seems content to remain in the fee-for-service world, essentially guaranteeing that innovation will come only from outside the industry. They seem to refuse to acknowledge the broad trends dominating most industries, including the move toward consumerism, the rapid change in business models, and the development of interoperable information systems or at least more readily available information. But perhaps even more important, they refuse to acknowledge that the new systems, designs, and approaches deliver higher-quality care to more people for less money.

> "The health-care system seems content to remain in the fee-for-service world."

Look at how the consumer has taken charge of the travel industry. In the past, airline employees and travel agents issued tickets for passengers. The airlines didn't realize that the system produced a bad experience for passengers, who had to wait in long lines and blamed the company anytime a ticketing agent made a mistake. Then the airlines adopted a self-service model, where passengers could book their travel,

144

get their ticket, and check in to their flight. The new system increased satisfaction and produced a better experience by enabling autonomy, control, and convenience. It also improved financial results, removing the need for additional staff performing this function. They did the unthinkable. They put their customers in charge, with, of course, some guidance from the software.

In terms of interoperability, consider how industries have embraced open information systems as a necessary condition. Take the banking industry as an example. Once upon a time, ATMs only worked for certain credit cards, and people spent time finding one that worked for them. This became a significant disruption to daily life, since most people only use ATMs when they have an immediate need for cash. Finally, the government stepped in and mandated all ATMs become interoperable, providing consumers greater access and availability no matter the credit card or ATM used. Overnight, the problem that had prevented people from getting the services and products they needed—when and where they needed them—vanished. The result? ATM use increased for everyone. The public benefitted. And the industry was allowed to charge for the added services, which created more revenue and also made them more efficient than the prior check writing/cashing system.

These examples make it clear why the current system is ripe for disruption. The historical pattern of every other industry is clear. The reluctance to develop new innovations only invites competitors with technological and business model expertise, untethered to the past and willing to experiment with new business models. The absence of providing real value to consumers creates the opportunity for others to fill that gap. And the lack of consumer convenience, access, transparency, and power only promises new innovations that upset the current system by fulfilling unsatisfied expectations. Consider Amazon, which is being asked to enter both the PBM and health-care businesses. Imagine the value they could bring through their capacity and capability for innovation and service. Look at what they are doing in and to retail. As I write, CVS Health is merging with Aetna, in part as a response to Amazon's likely entry into the health-care industry. Whether this move is right or wrong, it was reported that the company's management team presented approximately a dozen strategies to their board, and they considered the merger the best move to reinvent the company's future and serve their members.[29] This is a forward-looking company with a smart board of directors.

The system must wake up to a new reality that health care is fundamentally an information business focused on consumers. To ignore this reality means to follow the same path as other enterprises forced out of existence by companies that

---

[29] Sharon Terlep and Laura Stevens. "The Real Reason CVS Wants to Buy Aetna? Amazon," *The Wall Street Journal*, October 27, 2017, https://www.wsj.com/articles/the-real-reason-cvs-wants-to-buy-aetna-amazon-com-1509057307

recognized it. This means the health-care industry must adopt the innovation imperative and reinvent themselves, which consumers and large self-insured employers are demanding.

Health-care systems, hospitals, payers, PBMs, pharmaceutical companies, and physicians all need to think differently. Let's consider the new role each of these stakeholders must embrace in a consumer-driven, value-based model of care. Physicians need to embrace smart technologies (and we acknowledge, those are not today's EHRs) and must become counselors and navigators as well as healers. In this new role, they empower people to manage their health independently, while helping them find or prescribing the best solutions—whether drugs, exercise, nutrition, counseling, or simple information—and determine the best care available for their needs. This doesn't mean physicians no longer provide care; they do, except only for those aspects of health for which they have the time, capability, and

> "They empower people to manage their health independently, while helping them find or prescribing the best solutions."

capacity to improve. This new role calls for a far different perception of what it means to work as a physician, where volume no longer dictates decision making but rather what is valuable for the consumer.

Similarly, hospitals and health systems must also embrace

a more consumer-focused role rather than perceive their business as delivering as much care and service as possible and keeping every bed full. They must try to improve care using the least amount of resources and, when appropriate, refer people to the lowest cost alternative, which may include not just visiting another facility but receiving alternative forms of care—preventative physical therapy versus surgery, for example. Hospitals should also realize they are no longer geographically protected. Today, consumers continually demonstrate a willingness to travel across state lines to receive care.

And as informed, connected health consumers take over, they will shift the information balance and use the internet as not just an information tool but also as a diagnostic tool that can inform and direct care. A great example came from Dr. Lloyd Minor, dean of Stanford Medical School, who shared what was the most compelling story I've heard to describe what's happening today. In the past, diagnosis began with a trip to the physician's office, and the more serious the condition, the more likely a second or third trip to a specialist was to be expected. He described that even for rare medical issues, the internet has become an increasingly useful diagnostic tool,

148

> "Hospitals and health systems must also embrace a more consumer-focused role."

illustrating why patients are more frequently bringing the information—i.e., the diagnosis—to the physician rather than the other way around. Dr. Minor discovered a condition called superior semicircular canal dehiscence syndrome (SCDS). But like much of the exponentially growing information in medical science, the challenge was how to share that information with physicians. He tells the story, which was reported on ABC's *Medical Mysteries,* of a patient who relied on the health-care system for 22 years to identify and fix a medical problem he was having, with no success. Finally, after undergoing three operations for the wrong diagnosis, he consulted the internet and found the work Dr. Minor had pioneered and his discovery. He traveled from Germany to Johns Hopkins Medical Center in Baltimore to undergo a surgical procedure by Dr. Minor. Today, he is cured, all thanks to the power of the internet to share information.

149

Informed, connected health consumers begin their search on the internet as the first place to look for answers to their health questions. This is followed by checking with their family and friends, their pharmacist, their physician, and then the hospital. Consumers' willingness to travel for care, coupled with where they turn for information, means hospitals must increasingly stake out a different role—perhaps a specialized role where they can prove they deliver quality—and promote it actively via the internet. Why? On the one hand, hospitals must specialize in the services they perform often and well—versus making available anything the customer needs—to develop the expertise and capacity consumers would be willing to travel for. We've seen this all over as large department stores that have everything have been replaced with specialty stores that deliver a higher-quality, more informed experience. This will become increasingly important as generalized care becomes "outsourced" to consumers (think over-the-counter drugs but now with technology that allows consumers to handle basic care at home) as well as less expensive, more accessible community care providers or pharmacies with urgent care capacity.

Lowe's, one of the country's most innovative self-insured employers, tells its employees that they can go anywhere they want for heart surgery, but if they want Lowe's to cover the cost, they need to fly to the Cleveland Clinic. Lowe's doesn't send its employees to Cleveland Clinic for heart surgery because it performs a full spectrum of procedures. Rather, it chose Cleveland Clinic because it performs thousands of heart surgeries each year and can guarantee a level of quality other health-care providers simply can't. A heart surgery with complications is bad for the employee, bad for productivity, and very costly. So Lowe's agrees to cover the full cost of the procedure, including travel expenses for the patient and his or her significant other. Lowe's determined that it was less expensive to provide quality care the first time than deal with complications. And it's a big win for their employees. In the past, perhaps only the CEO could fly across the country for world-class care. Now, care has been democratized. Janitor or CEO, if you need heart surgery, it's world class. Higher quality, lower overall costs.

With specialization, hospitals must become more active in marketing and promoting their brand, leveraging the internet to educate consumers about the cost and quality of their services, and perhaps what those services are. A great example was my

"With specialization, hospitals must become more active in marketing and promoting their brand."

daughter's decision to have her knee surgery at the Steadman Clinic in Vail, Colorado. Despite living near four of the top health systems in the country, she chose to travel from Chicago for her procedure. Why? The Steadman Clinic offered her what other health-care providers didn't: clear information, education, quality metrics, and ultimately, a better experience. They treated her as an informed, connected health consumer rather than the patriarchal treatment she received from physicians and surgeons in Chicago, who, frankly, were not happy to be questioned about how many procedures they had performed and their quality, infection rates, and success rates. They will need to get used to that, particularly from women, who drive 80 percent of all health-care decisions.

But the need for innovation doesn't stop with health-care

providers. Payers also need to rethink and redefine themselves, starting with becoming more consumer focused. Aetna provides a good example. The health insurer hired former Harvard Business School professor Gary Loveman—who was most recently running Harrah's and Caesars casinos—to operate its health-care business. Why? What do business professors and casino professionals know about health care? Health care is fundamentally about consumers and changing behavior, and no one understands behavior better than casinos. Loveman's seminal article at Harvard, "Putting the Service-Profit Chain to Work," written in 1994, launched him into the world of behavior change. And Aetna knew that was what their business was really all about or at least headed in that direction. The smartest and most innovative payers understand they will need to invest in innovations that actually improve lifestyle behaviors and carve them out as a benefit, such as solutions that empower people to manage their health outside the constraints of the current system of care. They also need to focus on providing measurable value. Rather than send patients to the best health-care providers that are in their networks—where they benefit—they must send health consumers to the best destinations for care regardless of

"Health care is fundamentally about consumers and changing behavior."

their respective rebate and network relationships. And like hospitals, payers must also become more transparent around cost and quality because as their customers—in particular, large self-insured employers—become more knowledgeable about rebates and other practices, they are losing confidence that payers are truly on the same team. Finally, payers need to leverage the power of the internet to connect with and educate health consumers.

As pharmacy benefit managers (PBMs) increasingly find themselves under public scrutiny, they too must embrace a different role. This new role begins with shifting the focus to what provides long-term value for health consumers. When PBMs first began, they were all about providing medications at the lowest costs. Today, they provide a broader range of services, but many of their customers no longer believe they are providing the lowest-cost medication options to employers. Today, concerns have been raised that PBM practices drive up costs, limit access for certain patients, and decrease transparency. Rebates have become increasingly transparent and a big concern to those paying the bills. While these may work in the interim, they only spur political and health-consumer outrage, invite more government regulation, and open the door for others to provide more innovative solutions that offer value. Just like health-care providers and payers, PBMs must find ways to provide consumers with solutions that make it easier to stay healthy. And the leading PBMs are beginning to do just that—in a build, buy, or partnering mode with innovative companies that bring enhanced services focused on driving down cost and increasing quality and value. This is the direction that CVS is heading, changing its name to CVS Health, and recently announcing the acquisition of Aetna. Express Scripts is also introducing new models that focus on much more than the cost of medications.

> **"Pharma must begin to price for value and share in the savings delivered."**

Similarly, pharmaceutical companies also need to reimagine their role in the new health-care system of tomorrow. We believe that pharma, which today accounts for between 10 and 15 percent of health-care costs (a rate that is increasing),[30] is a key part of the solution for health and health care in the future—but only if they reinvent their model in three fundamental ways.

First, pharma must begin to price for value and share in the savings delivered. The best example is hepatitis C. Pharma found a cure, which is quite remarkable. But the drug cost, the way it is billed today, is too high for people and companies to afford. However, that line of thinking is only true if you look at the first year rather than cost avoidance over the patient's life. Over 10 years, curing someone today is not only a great

---

[30] "A Look at Drug Spending in the U.S." *The Pew Charitable Trusts*. Updated April 28, 2018. Accessed June 11, 2018. http://www.pewtrusts.org/en/research-and-analysis/fact-sheets/2018/02/a-look-at-drug-spending-in-the-us.

decision for their quality of life but a better clinical decision (less damage to other organs) and a better financial decision (less overall cost). So pharma needs to invent a financing model for certain drugs. That is not a nice-to-have; it's a requirement of their business.

Second, pharma needs to take responsibility for the full experience surrounding the drug, including adherence. They have to understand the health consumer and experience, and get someone to take the medication and continue to take it. This is good for the patient and good for pharma, as proper compliance could double their market size. Today, research shows that approximately half of all medications for chronic conditions are not taken as prescribed, and 20 to 30 percent of medication prescriptions are never filled.[31] The lack of medication adherence is estimated to cost the US health-care system between $100 and $289 billion.

Third, pharma needs to begin to be transparent about what medications work for whom. This will require them to be "smarter" about their business, with more studies—not clinical trials—based on real-world evidence. Lilly is leading the way here, focusing attention on what works in the market, how drugs are being used, and other factors. Similarly, when Abbott introduced its new Libre continuous glucose monitor, it brought to the FDA real-world evidence and studies on

[31] Meera Viswanathan, Carol E. Golin, Christine D. Jones, Mahima Ashok, Susan J. Blalock, Roberta C. M. Wines, Emmanuel J. L. Coker-Schwimmer, David L. Rosen, Priyanka Sista, Kathleen N. Lohr. "Interventions to improve adherence to self-administered medications for chronic diseases in the United States: a systematic review." *Annals of internal medicine.* December 04, 2012. Accessed January 21, 2018. https://www.ncbi.nlm.nih.gov/pubmed/22964778.

more than 100,000 users around the globe and received faster approval than expected. In addition, genetic and other testing to determine which drugs will work on which patients will be both necessary and required in our smarter future. These three requirements raise the bar significantly on what the current model asks of pharma but represent the new reality going forward. And while this seems like a lot of change, it will not only benefit pharma but is the only way for it to survive.

So if innovation is imperative, where do we begin? I like to say that "innovation begins by doing something," so the industry must begin to embrace innovation as a core element rather than a "pilot" or an "experiment." The most innovative self-insured employers have taken matters into their own hands—not content or willing to wait any longer—and started to partner with newer, more innovative companies that offer improved satisfaction of their employees, measurable clinical outcomes, and strong financial results. These large self-insured employers recognize the value of combining the advantage of scale with entrepreneurial companies' advantage in innovation. By entrepreneurial companies, I mean those with technological, process, and service innovations that make information and addressing the needs of health consumers

> **"The most innovative self-insured employers have taken matters into their own hands."**

central to their core value propositions. In health care, these companies offer solutions that empower people to better manage their individual conditions

"We can scale innovations that make a difference in health by combining small and large for short-term and long-term results and success."

but do so across entire populations. That scale feeds back into the systems, enabling these newer, entrepreneurial companies to have network effects on their data science and generate even better information.

What these newer, smaller entrepreneurial companies lack, large companies provide in abundance. Self-insured employers bring their workforce, payers bring the populations they insure, health systems bring the patients they care for, and PBMs bring the customers they serve. We can scale innovations that make a difference in health by combining small and large for short-term and long-term results and success. Over time, the value of this model only increases, as more people using the innovation means more information, which equals more precise knowledge.

Combining in this sense doesn't mean acquiring. Plenty of large companies attempt to innovate by acquiring smaller, more innovative enterprises, only to dampen the innovation. The newly acquired companies accept new policies, procedures, and cultural norms that are foreign to them and different from

157

what fueled their innovation in the first place. Inevitably, many acquisitions allow the scale of their acquirers to overpower and eventually overwhelm the company and the innovation by removing the boundaries that protect its integrity. In this context, scale always wins over innovation, never the other way around. Consider how hard it becomes for any large company to innovate on a sizable scale. It took IBM years to shake its successful and market-dominant mainframe approach. While once a strength, it became a weakness as the new environment demanded innovation, and IBM struggled to overcome

> "Rather than view innovation as a one-time event, we must embrace it as an ongoing cycle."

resistance from employees deeply invested in the status quo. Large companies are simply not good at innovating; rather, they're good at providing the products and services that made them established enterprises in the first place. Even Google today struggles with its size as a challenge to innovation and has even reorganized to try to protect and promote its creative spark.

So what does this mean? Thomas Edison offered a great quote after inventing the light bulb. He said of his many previous attempts, "I didn't fail. I just found a thousand ways that didn't work." Rather than view innovation as a one-time event, we must embrace it as an ongoing cycle that requires not only introducing new solutions but also testing, evaluating, and improving them. It means those within the health-care system must answer today's call for change. The best way to change is to look beyond the decades-old system to those who understand information and consumers best. These companies will enter the health-care equation, whether the players who are currently entrenched in the traditional health-care system like it or not. To perpetuate the status quo only means to ignore that innovation is not only inevitable but also encroaching on the existing model every day in a hundred ways. Amazon knows this. Apple knows this. Plenty of today's most information-and-consumer-minded companies understand it. It's time for the health-care system to grasp it too. They should accept that innovation is necessary and partner with those who can bring them into the new models | 159 of health care—before it's too late.

As my friend Jeff Salz likes to say, "It's time for everyone to leap before they look."

• • •

Chapter Summary

- "They [traditional health-care players] seem to refuse to acknowledge the broad trends dominating most industries, including the move toward consumerism, the rapid change in business models, and the development of interoperable information systems or at least more readily available information. But perhaps even more important, they refuse to acknowledge that the new systems, designs, and approaches deliver higher-quality care to more people for less money."

- "I like to say that 'innovation begins by doing something,' so the industry must begin to embrace innovation as a core element rather than a 'pilot' or an 'experiment.'"

- "The most innovative self-insured employers have taken matters into their own hands—not content or willing to wait any longer—and started to partner with newer, more innovative companies that offer improved satisfaction of their employees, measurable clinical outcomes, and strong financial results. These large self-insured employers recognize the value of combining the advantage of scale with entrepreneurial companies' advantage in innovation."

CONCLUSION

"If you are deliberately trying to create a future that feels safe, you will willfully ignore the future that is likely."

—Judith McNaught

Empowering individuals is the only viable and sustainable solution to successfully managing chronic conditions. The empowerment process begins by giving informed, connected health consumers the information and tools they need to manage their condition on their terms, not on ours. To understand why empowerment serves as the only path forward, consider what it means to live with a chronic condition. As a leading expert on behavioral issues related to diabetes, Dr. William Polonsky describes the experience of living with Type 1 or Type 2 Diabetes—which we can expand to include other chronic conditions—as follows: "Imagine the universe handed you another job you didn't ask for and certainly didn't want. A job without vacation . . . without pay . . . one you can't refuse . . . and one you're not even sure how to do right." Now, ask yourself, does a job with no time off and no pay sound "engaging"? How would you feel if someone regularly called asking you to spend more time on that job? Now, imagine someone gave you the tools to effectively manage that job and spend less time doing it. They wouldn't have to convince you to use those tools. You would understand immediately the value and how the tools empowered you to take charge of your life and condition. This is what informed, connected health consumers are demanding. They want to become empowered to live beyond the shadow of their chronic conditions.

Empowerment calls for three fundamental components. The first, and most important, starts with informed, connected health consumers and how we equip them to become both more informed and more in control of their health using real-time information that is personalized, context aware, simple, and actionable. "Personalized" means tailored to them, not someone else—a solution designed specifically for your *body's vital narrative.* "Context aware" recognizes that what works only does so at a certain place and time. "Simple" means a solution that not only eliminates the hassle map we are all so familiar with in health care but is also easy to use, ideally without any specialized training, and makes it easier to stay healthy. "Actionable" calls for information you can use in the moment that propels you to the goal, which is a better and healthier life. Think "bite-sized"—not a full meal. Today, fewer and fewer people have time for a full meal when it comes to using health-care solutions.

Informed, connected health consumers also want to be, as the name implies, connected. As we have more and more time in front of computers, we'll find that staying healthy requires more contact with people—real people. And this is even more true with chronic conditions. People with chronic conditions will want a connected community of people sharing their experiences, curated to just what they want and need. A community that not only provides caring support to help physiological health but psychological and social health as well. The caring community offers the greatest indicator of how well people manage their chronic conditions. In a soon-to-be-published study of people enrolled in the Livongo Diabetes Program, Dr. Jennifer Schneider and her team of researchers and data scientists found that people who share their blood glucose testing results better manage their conditions after 12 to 15 months than people who do not share. A simple but very important conclusion. We need to understand that chronic conditions and their successful management are more than physiological—they are psychosocial. When informed, connected health consumers surround themselves with people all striving toward the same goal—staying healthy—they are far more likely to achieve that objective.

Importantly, informed, connected health consumers want to control their own care. Even with access to information and a caring community, people with chronic conditions need assistance when their conditions prevent them from self-management. Real-time, context-aware care comes in the form of remote support from trained specialists and in-person assistance from members of the personal care team who can provide physical care. Care, in this model, no longer means physicians or hospitals. Rather, it means whatever people need to optimize their health in the moment, whether information, encouragement, or simply a helping hand. But people still want to set the standards for what care is delivered, by whom, and when it is provided. We may disagree with those standards, but it's their life, their health, and their decision—and should not and will not be determined by a doctor, a payer, or a hospital.

164

It's about trusting that we, in fact, can make the best decisions about our own health with the right information and about giving us that opportunity. Trusting that each of us can make the right decision about our own health care and do so on our terms is a fundamental tenet of this book.

These three components reflect the behavioral journey informed, connected health consumers are beginning, to improve their health. This path exists outside the traditional "health-care" system of physicians, hospitals, and payers. For the first time, we can and will truly empower people with chronic conditions and make it easier for them to live better and healthier lives. The journey starts with health consumers seeking information to answer their questions (i.e., self-diagnosing via the internet). When they lack information, they seek advice from their caring community (i.e., health forums, family, and friends). And when they need help, they will seek services (more often in forms that exclude a traditional doctor's visit). Naturally, we must build a model that not only supports these behaviors but also enhances them to meet a new level of needs, expectations, and measurable clinical and financial results.

Our research and experience, at Livongo and many other places, demonstrate that this way to health is a better model for improving satisfaction, clinical outcomes, and financial results, which is all that really matters. And every day, we're learning from our members, our clients, and our own data scientists.

As PepsiCo, Iron Mountain, and WEA Trust demonstrate, there is no single path to innovation, only the need to embrace it as an imperative and keep learning. Coming in a variety of forms, innovation revolves around the health consumer, the effort to become more accountable and smarter for how we use resources, and the push to leverage information as an inexpensive, effective, and sustainable resource. PepsiCo, Iron Mountain, and WEA Trust are taking different approaches to personalizing solutions for their respective populations, yet they are following the same fundamental model by leveraging their scale with smaller, innovative companies that can drive significant value. All continue to achieve improved measurable outcomes in terms of cost, quality of care, and satisfaction— and the journey is only beginning.

166

We have made considerable progress in recent years in addressing chronic conditions with effective solutions, but our most important work remains. We must continue our commitment toward putting the informed, connected health consumer at the center of the experience to drive better outcomes. And then we must trust them with the most important thing in the world: their health and the health of those they love. But in the end, it's not our choice. Health consumers want to own the responsibility for their health. And they are demanding it. And we should too.

CITATIONS

2014 Physician Specialty Data Book. Washington, DC: Association of Medical Colleges, June 3, 2015.

"6 Lessons from Pepsi on Engaging Employees beyond Workplace Wellness." *Engaging Leader.* April 28, 2016. http://www.engagingleader.com/6-lessons-from-pepsi/

"A Look at Drug Spending in the U.S." *The Pew Charitable Trusts.* Updated April 28, 2018. Accessed June 11, 2018. http://www.pewtrusts.org/en/research-and-analysis/fact-sheets/2018/02/a-look-at-drug-spending-in-the-us.

Adams, Kelly M., W. Scott Butsch, and Martin Kohlmeier. "The State of Nutrition Education at US Medical Schools." *Journal of Biomedical Education* 2015 (August 06, 2015): http://dx.doi.org/10.1155/2015/357627

Alonso-Zaldivar, Ricardo, and Kevin S. Vineys. "AP Count: Nearly 11.8M Enroll for Obama Health Law in 2018." AP News. February 07, 2018. Accessed May 29, 2018. https://www.apnews.com/837a78792b944937b6e0fca69ee55e4e/AP-count:-Nearly-11.8M-enroll-for-Obama-health-law-in-2018.

"At a Glance 2015." National Center for Chronic Disease Prevention and Health Promotion. Accessed September 13, 2017. https://www.cdc.gov/chronicdisease/resources/publications/aag/pdf/2015/nccdphp-aag.pdf

Banerji, Mary Ann, and Jeffrey D. Dunn. "Impact of Glycemic Control on Healthcare Resource Utilization and Costs of Type 2 Diabetes: Current and Future Pharmacologic Approaches to Improving Outcomes." *American Health & Drug Benefits* 6, no. 7 (September 2013), 382-392, Accessed September 13, 2017. https://www.ncbi.nlm.nih.gov/pmc/articles/PMC4031727/

168

Beals, Rachel Koning. "Chicago cab report shows fast-approaching demise at hands of Uber and Lyft." *MarketWatch*. June 06, 2017. Accessed October 2, 2017. http://www.marketwatch. com/story/chicago-cab-report-shows-fast-approaching-demise-at-hands-of-uber-and-lyft-2017-06-06

Buttorff, Christine, Teague Ruder, and Melissa Bauman. *Multiple Chronic Conditions in the United States*. Santa Monica: RAND Corporation, 2017.

"Chronic Disease Prevention and Health Promotion." Centers for Disease Control and Prevention. Last modified December 18, 2017. Accessed January 25, 2018. https://www.cdc.gov/chronicdisease/index.htm

Coleman, Jackie, and John Coleman. "Increase the Odds of Achieving Your Goals by Setting Them with Your Spouse." *Harvard Business* Review. February 3, 2015. Accessed June 11, 2018. https://hbr.org/2015/02/increase-the-odds-of-achieving-your-goals-by-setting-them-with-your-spouse

"Cuba." The World Bank Group. Accessed September 26, 2017. https://data.worldbank.org/country/cuba?view=chart

C. William Keck, and Gail A. Reed. "The Curious Case of Cuba." *American Journal of Public Health* 102, no. 8 (August 2012), Accessed June 6, 2018. DOI: 10.2105/AJPH.2012.300822

Downing, Janelle, Jenna Bollyky, and Jennifer Schneider. "Use of a Connected Glucose Meter and Certified Diabetes Educator Coaching to Decrease the Likelihood of Abnormal Blood Glucose Excursions: The Livongo for Diabetes Program." *Journal of Medical Internet Research* 19, no.7 (July 2017), Accessed August 14, 2017. DOI: 10.2196/jmir.6659

"Fitbit invests $6M in glucose monitoring startup Sano."
MobiHealthNews. January 08, 2018. Accessed January 15, 2018.
http://www.mobihealthnews.com/content/fitbit-invests-6m-
glucose-monitoring-startup-sano

From the Ground Up. Boston: Iora Health, 2016. Accessed November
8, 2017. http://online.pubhtml5.com/lcuv/bkxo/

Kanthawala, Shaheen, Amber Vermeesch, Barbara Given, and Jina
Huh. "Answers to Health Questions: Internet Search Results
Versus Online Health Community Responses." *Journal of
Medical Internet Research* 18, no. 4 (April 2016), 95, Accessed
September 28, 2017. DOI:10.2196/jmir.5369

Livongo Clinical and Financial Outcomes Report. Mountain View:
Livongo Health, June 2016. Accessed August 14, 2017. https://
www.livongo.com/docs/pdf/Livongo%20Clinical%20and%20
Financial%20Outcomes%20Report.pdf

"Livongo Net Promoter Score from Member Satisfaction Survey."
Livongo Health, September 2016.

Lupkin, Joshua. "Taxis, Liveries, and Limousines." *Encyclopedia of
Chicago*. Accessed September 28, 2017. http://www.encyclope-
dia.chicagohistory.org/pages/1232.html

"Statistics About Diabetes." *American Diabetes Association*. Last
modified July 19, 2017. Accessed September 26, 2017. http://
www.diabetes.org/diabetes-basics/statistics/

Terlep, Sharon, and Laura Stevens. "The Real Reason CVS Wants to Buy Aetna? Amazon." *The Wall Street Journal*. October 27, 2017. Accessed November 3, 2017. https://www.wsj.com/articles/the-real-reason-cvs-wants-to-buy-aetna-amazon-com-1509057307

The world health report 1997 - conquering suffering, enriching humanity. Geneva: The World Health Organization, 1997. http://www.who.int/whr/1997/en/

Viswanathan, Meera, Carol E. Golin, Christine D. Jones, Mahima Ashok, Susan J. Blalock, Roberta C. M. Wines, Emmanuel J. L. Coker-Schwimmer, David L. Rosen, Priyanka Sista, Kathleen N. Lohr. "Interventions to improve adherence to self-administered medications for chronic diseases in the United States: a systematic review." *Annals of internal medicine*. December 04, 2012. Accessed January 21, 2018. https://www.ncbi.nlm.nih.gov/pubmed/22964778

World Health Organization: Adherence to long-term therapies. Evidence for action. Geneva: World Health Organization, 2003. http://www.who.int/chp/knowledge/publications/adherence_full_report.pdf?ua=1